Body Brilliance

The 8 Royal Diamonds

For A Healthier and More Radiant You

Rino Soriano

Disclaimer

This book is designed to provide information on holistic health living. It is distributed with the understanding that the author and publisher are not engaged in rendering medical advice or medical claims about your health and well-being. Rino is not a licensed health practitioner. He is a holistic chef, certified fitness trainer, certified sports nutritionist and educator in holistic health and has experience in holistic nutrition, fitness, and supplemental health programs. If medical advice is required, the services of a qualified healthcare practitioner should be sought. Every effort has been made to make this manual complete and as accurate as possible. However, there may be errors in both typographical and content. Therefore, this text should be used as a general guide and not the ultimate source for improving your health. Furthermore, this manual contains holistic health information that is current only up to the printing date.

The main intent of this manual is to educate and entertain. Body Brilliance and the author shall have neither liability nor responsibility to any person or entity with respect to any loss or damage caused by or allegedly to have been caused, directly or indirectly, by using the information in this book.

Table of Contents

Message From The Author

Hi, I want you to know that I wrote this book from my heart to help clarify and simplify the topic of health and wellness. I do not claim to be an expert that wants you to follow every word I say. I am here to present to you sound holistic habits and perspectives that in turn shall help you to look at your life and your health from a Higher point of view. You are unique in mind, body and spirit so you require to honor and take into consideration your uniqueness. This shall then be able to help you to determine what life environment will help you to create the optimal conditions for your health and wellness and your Higher Potential. It is my sincere desire for you to create optimum health, wellness and achieve your Highest Potential. I pray that my book at the very least sparks you to remembering who you truly are.

Happy Learning and Happy Body Brilliance.

Rino Soriano

Chapter 1

The Multiple Dimensions of Health

When people hear the term "health," they typically think that it mainly involves how they feel and what they are putting into their bodies via foods and beverages. This narrow perspective of health is the cause of why so many do not fully comprehend the full aspect of what health really is. So, what is health really and what are the true dynamics involved?

In essence, your health is multi-dimensional and incorporates many aspects of your life from the foods you eat, the work you do and even down to the smell of your home. These are all impacting your health to some degree. Even the people you live with are directly affecting your health every day, whether you aware of this or not.

At the fundamental level of life, your health is being affected by everything you come into contact with, wherever you are, at any given time. Have you ever walked into someone's home and it smelled dank or foul? How did you feel in that moment? How about when walking into a person's home where there is clutter everywhere. How did you feel then? What about when a person that you really enjoy being around walked into the room? How did you feel inside?

My point is that everything in your life and every circumstance that occurs will impact your health at some level. So, perhaps the time has come for a new perspective on your health and what exactly that entails. It may serve you well to begin to awaken to the fact that your health and your whole life are interconnected at all levels. The décor in your home and the colors you have around your rooms are also impacting your health. Even the amount of sunlight coming in through your windows is impacting your health.

I think by now you get the idea that your health involves so much more than how you feel, how you look and what you eat on a daily basis. Even the music you listen to can profoundly affect how you feel and does impact your health. Essentially, my message is to teach you or more specifically awaken you to a Higher level of Truth in regards to your health.

With this new awareness you can now elevate your life so that it, in turn, impacts your health in very beneficial ways. Imagine if each decision you require to make in your life takes into consideration how it will affect your health? This is a very powerful perspective and I believe is the only way that you can truly get to the level of health you really desire.

Imagine for a moment if you felt absolutely fantastic every day of your life. Imagine having a radiant glow about you and a feeling of youthfulness and vitality. Imagine your life living in this state of being. What do you think you could accomplish and how much would you appreciate your life even more feeling and looking fantastic at this optimal state of being? You can experience this, my friend, you really can! With the proper guidance and information you can feel and look better than you ever have in your entire life.

Are you ready for this Higher level of Truth and of living? If you are then you are about to embark on one amazing journey. You see, it is only through self- empowerment can you attain this optimum state of health and wellbeing. It is time to assume your power and discover a Higher level of Truth. This will benefit everyone and everything on this planet. **Happy Health Journey!**

Chapter 2

Your Body Is Programmed For Perfect Health

Did you know that every single cell in your body is programmed for perfect health? It's true. This means that you have the potential to feel great almost every single day of your life. This program for perfect health is fixed into your DNA. What science has discovered is that because of this blueprint for perfect health in your cells, the body can restore itself from any injury, disorder, or chronic illness. The body has a divine mechanism that senses when there is an injury or disequilibrium in your body. As such, your body knows exactly how to restore itself back to its divine perfection.

To illustrate the divine capability of the human body, let's use an example that we all have experienced. You have probably cut yourself numerous times throughout your life, correct? As is the normal case, your body healed that cut within seven to ten days depending upon the severity of the wound.

Did you know that the second you get cut or receive any injury for that matter, your brain immediately senses this trauma and begins sending all the appropriate compounds to the injury site to heal it? This all happens unconsciously and without you having to add a thing to the wound. Again, there is a program in your cells for this to occur automatically. Is this amazing or what? Typically, your wound heals completely within a couple weeks and most of the time you can't even tell you had a cut.

When you put something in your body that is foreign or synthetic, it causes your cells to produce toxins which in turn affects your organs and suppresses your immune system. This is exactly what synthetic compounds and drugs do to your bodily systems; they create a polluted internal environment which opens the doorway to organ failure and chronic illness. The body can produce its own healing compounds in the form of natural bio-chemicals. These are the most powerful compounds in helping the body to heal. Your cells don't want anything synthetic that act as poisons in your system. This only makes the body's job harder.

The body is an immaculate creation. It is a perfect creation. It knows how to heal itself. Look at the facts and you will see the truth. When you get a cut or break a bone or worse, the body heals it every time. It is guaranteed to be effective and perfect in every case. Again, look at your life and how many times you have received injuries. Your body restored every single wound and trauma. Your body can also heal any disease using this same divine mechanism.

If the body is programmed for perfect health then why are you and so many people sick and tired? This is the million dollar question. Yet, there is a simple explanation. You see, when you step outside of what nature has set before you, this is when you run into problems. Nature is perfect and supplies all of the inhabitants of this planet with their needs, people and animals alike. Where things go awry is when someone or something attempts to mess with the divineness of nature. This is exactly what man has done over the years. Man has attempted to alter and manipulate what nature has given. This is wrong and can only lead to major complications, as is evident with what is transpiring in the world today.

Despite all the advancements in technology and improvements in general living, the average person is not even close to feeling optimally healthy.

Nature knows best and holds the keys to optimum health. The answers to optimum health are always and will always be found in nature. Your body is designed to be nourished from natural foods and ingredients. It is just like when you put gas in your car. Put the right kind of gas in your tank and your car runs perfectly. Put the wrong kind of gas in there and now you have problems.

Genetically modified foods, processed foods, micro-waved foods and foods that are loaded with chemicals and toxins are not meant to go in the body and as such causes the body to malfunction. Grocery stores are loaded with foods that are so chemically altered from their natural form. When you deviate from nature in this aspect, it is only a matter of time before serious complications arise, as is evident with the health of most people across the globe. In fact, there is an epidemic at hand which is growing every year.

The solution to all this is to go back to nature. This is the key and is the only way to optimum health. Nature holds all the solutions to your health and wellbeing. Did you know that Mother Earth nourishes you with vital energy? In fact, without receiving this healing energy on a continual basis, you would die. Astronauts at times get very sick when they are up in space because they are not receiving this healing energy. Next time you are not feeling well or feel weak and tired, go in your back yard and lay in the grass face down for ten minutes and notice how you feel. It will energize you and invigorate your being.

Here is a little secret of why so many people enjoy the beach and being near bodies of water: First of all, the beach is a place where negative ions are in abundance. Ions energize your body and can even elevate your mood to one of happiness and joy from the impact they have on your brain's neurotransmitters. Also, the beach contains sand which is literally crushed small crystals. Crystals emit healing energies that can transmute negative energies and can aid in healing the body. Crystals can also energize you and help you to feel alive. Now do you understand why the beach and other bodies of water are so healing? Another interesting fact is that when ocean waves crash up on the shore, there is a mist that is produced. In this natural process, the sea minerals in the water get aerosolized into the air and when you breathe them in you are nourishing your whole body. Is this great stuff or what?

Ions are also abundant in forests and the mountains. These outdoor places produce these negatively charged molecules naturally. These ions have been studied and researched extensively and are found to be extremely powerful healing compounds for the body and overall wellbeing.

Do you see the power of nature? Do you see how nature holds the solutions to most of the health issues of today? Yes, you must go back to nature as was intended. To continue at the current rate of our society will only lead to more disease and suffering for many people. You can't trick the body. It is highly intelligent and conscious. In fact, it knows more than you do. Learn to listen to your body and hear its messages to you. It is your best friend, treat it as such.

Holistic Living Practice:

Whenever you feel down and out, tired or depressed go out in nature somewhere. Go for a hike, a walk on the beach, a walk through the forest or simply lay in your backyard in the grass. This is an all-natural therapy for mind, body and spirit. Try it and see. You will be surprised at the results.

Your Body Is Highly Intelligent & Knows How To Heal Itself. You Just Have To Come To This Realization!

Chapter 3

Are You Out of Gas?

Let me begin by saying that when you boil everything down to the simplest of principles, you always have the truth sitting right there in front of you. Society has made such a game at converting all aspects of life into complexities that confuse people to the point where they are deceived and far from the truth. In the aspect of health, again, there is misinformation, deceit and pure fraud all in the name of POLITICS.

You see, creating optimum health is quite easy once you know the truth. You cannot create optimum health when you have information that is either deceiving or misinforming. The same way a roadmap gets you to your desired destination, so too does an optimum health roadmap get you to a healthy state of being.

You have been brainwashed with health information that does not help you to be optimally healthy. How can I say this? EASY…I live by a simple saying and that is…The Proof Is In The Pudding! Here is a secret that you can count on 100% of the time and you can use this little gem for all aspects of your life. It will always lead you in the right direction. **Life Will Always Reveal The Truth To You.**

The universe is always revealing the truth to you. Since you have been conditioned with so many lies and deceptions throughout your life, you cannot see the truth sitting right there in front of you. So, let's use this life principle in the aspect of optimum health.

If we simply take a look at our society and the health of the people in it, then we can clearly see that the information that has been presented to you over the years obviously lacks substance. If this information that has been taught to you and is available in mainstream society has any truth to it, don't you think we would have a much healthier group of people? Don't you think we would have many people being healthy and happy? Wouldn't we have people that look alive and vibrant?

The reality is quite the opposite. Millions of people are sick in one way or another. We have a society of tired, stressed out, depressed & overweight individuals. One out of two people are becoming chronically sick in this day and age of technology. One out of two people are overweight. I could go on and on with statistics of how this society is quite ill and not just in the body. Many people are ill in the mind as well.

It boggles my mind how our society doesn't see the epidemic of poor health that is present right in front of their eyes. So many people accept what they see on TV and read in the paper as true. You have been given a BIG HEAP of fraudulent information over the years all in the name of profit. The amount of deception that is present is mind boggling. Here is the reality…because you have been so conditioned since you were a child with misinformation, you cannot see the truth of life because you think this truth is wrong or twisted.

Again, I let life prove to me what is true and what is not. The truth is that most of the health information available in our society will not help you to create optimum health. Again, look at the facts and what is transpiring with the health of people in general. Look at yourself! Can you honestly say that feel optimally healthy? Be Honest! If you truly want to experience optimum health then is essential for you to empower yourself with information that serves you well. You have to become your own master and discover your truth from within.

The time has come where you have to make a decision. What is that decision? It is time to make a decision of whether you will continue to allow yourself to be conditioned with misinformation or whether you choose to empower yourself and take control of your own health. Again, life will always reveal the truth to you. Optimally healthy people are self-empowered from within and are vibrant and have excess energy. You have this potential as well. You were born to be optimally health. It is literally programmed into your cells. However, creating optimum health is a choice. The question is…WHAT DO YOU CHOOSE?

Why You And So Many People Feel Drained and Fatigued?

I always boil everything down to the simplest of principles. In fact, most of life is simple yet we have been conditioned to make things complex. So, let's look at the true reasons why you and so many people feel and look fatigued. This is easy to understand and yet you may be baffled and think that it must be some mysterious reason why you feel the way you do. Here we go… The following are the simple reasons why you and so many people feel tired all the time:

1) Cellular Dehydration

2) Nutrient Deficiencies

3) Oxygen Deficient

4) Deficiency in Essential Fatty Acids

5) Deficiency in Digestive & Metabolic Enzymes

6) Deficiency in Anti-Oxidant Levels

7) Pollution

8) EMF Frequencies in Abundance in the Environment

9) Unhealthy & Genetically Modified Food

10) Toxic Water

11) Polluted Air

12) Lack of Sunlight

13) Stress

There is nothing mysterious about why some people feel so fatigued and drained of energy all the time. Everything in life operates through simple principles or what some term science. There is a science to how everything runs, from your car to your radio to even how your body functions. In order for you to feel great you have to follow the simple science of how your body and cells operate.

Your car requires gas, oil and spark plugs to run; so too does your body require specific compounds in order for it to function properly. You wouldn't put milk in the gas tank of your car, would you? How about putting some chlorine in there? Or what about some liquid tar? You wouldn't put these compounds in there because they do not cause your car to run and in fact can damage your car tremendously, correct?

You probably ingest compounds on a daily basis that don't belong in your body. The human body is designed to run perfectly day in and day out. Your cells can only recognize and absorb specific foods, nutrients and oils. Most of the foods that are available at the market are either synthetically made or contain so many chemicals that your body does not recognize what it is let alone assimilate it.

The ironic thing that really baffles me time and time again is that a majority of our society treat their cars better than they do their body. They put the highest octane gas in their car, get the oil changed every few months, spend hours washing and waxing and even pay thousands of dollars extra in order to get the sport wheels or the sunroof. Listen, I am not here to judge anyone or say that any of this is bad or wrong. My intention is to make you conscious that this kind of behavior and attitude is why you and so many people in this world don't feel optimally healthy.

Tally all the money you spend on your car every year…for gas, oil, insurance, cleaning and general maintenance and you are paying one large chunk of your income for a metal object that will eventually break down. Does this make any sense? To spend a small fortune on a piece of metal that will never give you anything in return! Why wouldn't you want to expend all this time, energy and money on something that is so much more important than a piece of metal? Your Body Is Your Temple! Why wouldn't you care for your body with this same attitude and spend extra money to ensure you feel and look good? In fact, for a fraction of the cost of what you pay to maintain and insure your car, you could easily create a level of health that would boggle your mind.

So, these are the big reasons why you may feel fatigued a majority of the time. The majority of compounds you are putting in your body cannot sustain the cells. Toxic and dead food equals toxic and dead cells. This is so simple and yet you may not see it. Your body runs via a perfect science. It requires nutrients, oxygen, essential fatty acids, antioxidants, water, and even sunlight. Most of the food you buy at a supermarket is dead and contains low levels of nutrients. The vegetables and fruits contain very little nutrients in them because modern agriculture methods have wiped out the living bacteria that are the creators of hundreds of life giving bio-nutrients that your body requires for optimum health. They also get sprayed with pesticides and fertilizers that impact your health negatively.

Science has proven that most of the food supply of today is deficient in nutrients. How can you expect your body to run on toxic and nutrient deficient food? Would you expect your car to run on liquid tar or anything else other than gas? Here is the simplicity of the epidemic that we are faced with. YOUR BODY IS RUNNING ON EMPTY! IT IS OUT OF GAS.

Unlike your car though, your body is an immaculate conception. It can adapt and create nutrients for you, however, only for so long. Once your reserves get used up then you are riding on fumes. This is where most people are at today; RIDING ON FUMES. Again, it is simple to understand when we boil it down yet society has done a number on programming people to think that feeling good every day is some complex process and is only available to a select few.

You are born to be optimally healthy…it is programmed in your DNA. Again, follow the simple science of how the body is designed and you will feel great. Go against what nature has set before you and now you're in for a long and bumpy ride. Remember when I said earlier that life will always reveal to you the truth. Look at nature, look at the animals; they follow the simple science of how their body is designed. All the secrets of life and your health are right there in front of your eyes every day. Yet you miss it because you are so programmed to go against what the creator has gifted you with.

You are born to be healthy, this is a certainty. Science has proven it many times over. It all boils down to a choice. Do you choose to feel great or will you choose to continue to follow information that is obviously worthless? It's all a choice and so is life. So, what do you choose?

Every Choice Has A Consequence. Choose Wisely!

Chapter 4

Health Facts & Health Wisdom

Demystifying The Myths of Life

I want to demystify a number of health myths that have been floating around out there for some time. These myths are actually causing people to be misinformed and limiting their efforts to create an optimum level of health. I want clarify for you so you have a better comprehension of what is Truth and what is erroneous that you require letting go of.

Are you ready to discover the greatest myths ever presented to you? Again, prepare yourself to shed these illusions as they are hindering your ability to create an optimal level of health. In fact, some of these myths have done more to keep you and other people unwell than to benefit your health. Here we go my friend, the funny myths are about to be exposed.

The Low Fat Myth

You probably may believe that it is healthy to eat a low fat diet and to limit your total fat intake each day, correct? Well, this is actually one of the greatest myths ever created. Many people have done a disservice to their health and their families by following this erroneous myth. Let me present some basic science facts for you so that you may learn to discern the Truth of this topic as it is crucial for you to know. Regardless of what has been presented to you on this topic, the simple holistic science fact is…**fat is the most essential nutrient your body requires for optimal health**. It is required for many processes in your body and is a precursor to hormone production.

What this means is that your body requires a consistent supply of the right kinds of fat in order for you to have the right hormone levels in your body, along with keeping your immune system strong and for skin, hair, eyes and brain health. If you reduce total fat from your diet, you are going to alter your hormone chemistry along with being deficient in essential fatty acids that are required for optimum biological processes. Thus you may experience improper health and functioning of your body.

Also, fats are the greatest source of energy. Do you comprehend what this means? It means that you will actually have greater energy levels if you consume healthy fats on a consistent basis. So, by consuming healthy levels of fat every day, you are easily increasing your energy levels. The myth that says that fat makes you fat is actually false and has been proven scientifically. Actually, healthy fats get converted into water and lipids, both of which your body uses as nutrition and hydration. Again, this is simple holistic science.

The Truth is by consuming healthy fats on a consistent basis you will actually moderate and improve your metabolism. This means that you will actually reduce weight or maintain a healthy weight level. **Fat does not make you fat.** Now if you are going to eat plain fat all day long then you may put some weight on but who is going to do that, honestly?

You can validate this simple Truth by embodying this information in your daily nutrition intake. Keep in mind that you require to ingest the right kinds of fats, not just any type. What has been discovered around the world is that the cultures that ingest moderate to high amounts of healthy fats are the healthiest people on the planet. Again, this is simple science and validates itself. The fats that are harming people are the altered and hydrogenated forms. These fats are quite toxic to the system and these are the oils that are causing improper health in many people. Hydrogenated oils are super high heated and altered from their natural composition. When you heat a compound, you alter it on a molecular level and thus create something new. In the aspect of oils, when they are heated they are changed and become toxic to your system. These oils are the ones to stay away from.

Thus, oils like margarine, vegetable oils, canola oil, corn oil and the whole list of altered oils are the ones to stay away from regardless of what you may think. Canola oil has been presented as a healthy oil. Well, if you do some research it has been discovered to be toxic over long term use. If you learn about where it comes from and how it is processed then the Truth is that it is not a healthy oil to consume. **The healthy oils are natural, unaltered and very**

healthy for your body. These fats include avocado, olive oil, grapeseed oil, coconut oil, walnut oil, almond oil and palm oil. Be aware that it is not healthy to cook with most oils from the fact that you alter the composition when you heat the oil.

So, my recommendation is to use steam, roasting, and grilling with a little water to cook your meals and then at the completion when your food is fully cooked after you take it off the heat, then add your oil. So, for example, if you make a soup, place all the ingredients into the pot with water and then cook it until the soup is done. Now add your oil and spices to flavor and add the healthy component of the fat. If you do require using oil to cook with, I recommend using coconut oil and grapeseed oil as these have high smoking points and can be used safely if you cook with them quickly. **Funny Myth #1 exposed and vaporized!** You may visit my website to learn more about my Body Brilliance Holistic Slimming Multi-Media Kit. You can also visit Amazon.com to view my book on Holistic Slimming if you desire.

The Cardiovascular Myth

Here is another funny myth that has been presented as Truth, however, does not validate itself. Engaging in cardiovascular endurance activities at high levels several times per week is not conducive to optimum health. You know the activities I am talking about…aerobics, running, marathons, treadmill, and other activities and sports that result is extended elevation of heart levels. Let me clarify. Your body is equipped with some Divine capabilities and with reserve systems that help it to function and repair. The main point here is that if you engage in high intensity cardiovascular activities on a routine basis, you are actually depleting your body and your reserves to adequately repair and regenerate.

The current health paradigm is teaching you to go out 3 to 5 days a week at 45 minutes to 1 hour to do cardio activities. It is recommended to go at 60 to 75% of maximum heart rate capability. This is ludicrous to say the least. Where this came from I have no idea but let me give you a good example of what this philosophy is saying. Essentially, it is like running your car at 75% of its maximum capability on a consistent basis. It is like stomping on the gas pedal at a stop light to go every time. Or, another example is if you have a manual stick shift car, it is like driving your car using first and second gear only with revving the engine on a daily basis at high RPM levels. Do you think you car's engine will last long by running it in this manner? In fact, by doing this, the engine will burn out much faster.

Well, this is what people are doing to themselves by engaging in high intensity and long duration cardiovascular activities. Essentially, they are elevating their heart levels too high and potentially causing themselves harm over the long term. In fact, if you want to shorten your life span then this is one way to do that. So, the main point is, it is not healthy to engage in high intensity long duration activities and also unnecessary. Your heart doesn't require this type of stimulation to be healthy. Yes, you require being active, you just need to do it in a healthy manner. In fact, it is best to keep your heart rate at low to moderate levels when engaging in sport activities. This is why lifting weights in the right manner is the greatest activity you can do for looking and feeling your best. By lifting weights properly and for the right duration, you do so many awesome things for your health.

First, your body will produce many life regenerating hormones that will keep you young looking and feeling young. Second, you will put on muscle mass which in turn will help to keep your weight healthy by moderating your metabolism and you get the benefit of looking awesome. How amazing that a simple activity like lifting weights can do so many awesome things for your health. This is the #1 activity to engage in if you want to add many years to your life. There are also other processes going on with working out with weights as in strengthening your ligaments and tendons and also mental and emotional components that most people have no clue that comes from lifting weights. Again, you require to lift weights in the right manner otherwise, you are wasting time, money and energy. I can show anyone how to do it in the right manner. It is actually so simple yet most people are unaware.

What they teach at the gym, well, this is not very effective for most people because it is over working your muscles and then the nutrition habits of most people does not support maximum gains in health and building muscle. I will now give you a simple example that shall help you to see the Truth of how high endurance long duration activities are not healthy. If you simply observe the difference between a marathon runner and a sprinter the Truth becomes quite apparent. Whom do you think is healthier and has a better functioning body? The Truth is that the sprinter is way healthier than the marathon runner. In fact, not even close. The marathon runner is depleted and week compared to the sprinter. The marathon runner's activity and lifestyle don't allow for the body to recuperate or regenerate so thus they are in a catabolic (weak, degenerating) state.

In essence, their training and their activity is too depleting on the body and is never allowed to recuperate properly, thus simply looking at them will tell the tale and the Truth of the matter. The sprinter on the other hand is in anabolic phase and as is quite evident by simply observing their body, they are quite healthy looking and feeling. These athletes have high power, strength and musculature. Their body is in anabolic phase meaning they are regenerating and building muscle on a routine basis. Their activity is short duration and so is their training. This is the key and one of the main secrets for engaging in fitness activities.

You see, the body absolutely requires to be worked out, however, you require to do it in the right manner otherwise it has the opposite effect. Your muscles and body have only so many available nutrients, hydration and ATP energy to perform in activities. The intention is to engage in activities where you are using readily available bio-nutrients that your body has to give. You want to avoid engaging in either long duration sports or activities or high intensity activities that cause you to dip into your reserve supply of energy and nutrients. This is why most athletes have short careers because they consistently place their body into tapping into reserves and they never allow their body to recuperate adequately.

The main key is to engage in activities that are short duration or start stop sports. Sports like tennis, volleyball, lifting weights, pilates, hiking, power walking and other similar short duration or start stop activities are ideal for optimal health. These activities do not cause your body to dip into reserves as much as other sports. The other main key is to fully allow the body to recuperate after engaging in your activity. The secret is you can actually get in better shape by let's say working out with weights for only 25 to 30 minutes than if you spend 1 hour or more as most people do. In fact, the results are quite amazing when you see someone who does the proper weight training program as I teach, and the results they get with actually doing less.

So, my main point to you is…yes engage in activities and do them on a consistent basis, however, reduce the sports that will deplete you. Also, remember to allow full recovery after your sports.. Most people do not know how to do this properly. This is important if you want to regenerate and extend your life span. It is important to structure your nutrition intake as to replenish and regenerate your body properly along with using the right supplements for muscle recovery. As shall be presented throughout this book, you will be given the keys on how to do this more efficiently as to maximize results.

The Cholesterol Myth

In recent years there has been talk about cholesterol and how you need to limit total levels every day for better health. Really? No thanks…just another funny myth my friend! Here is another lie that has no scientific basis whatsoever. Once again, people have done themselves a great disservice by following such erroneous myths. Pay attention because I keep things very simple. Cholesterol is a required compound for optimum health. You need to ingest it in sufficient levels to maintain proper functioning of your body. It has numerous functions to keeping you young looking, vital and feeling healthy. The simple fact is, if you ingest the right kinds of fats then you will receive the healthy cholesterol type that benefits your health and longevity. If you do not ingest the right kind of cholesterol then you are doing yourself a disservice.

In fact some people who have reduced their overall cholesterol in their diet actually got high cholesterol a few months after engaging in such a lifestyle. So, what is the Truth then? Well, if you use the life philosophy of Life Will Always Reveal The Truth To You, then you know what is a funny myth and what is of Truth.

The harmful cholesterol only comes from hydrogenated oils and fats that are chemically altered from their natural state. So, the key is to eat the right kinds of oils and fats and do it on a consistent basis. You won't have to ever worry about getting high cholesterol levels because your body will moderate it just fine because you are ingesting the right fats. If you ingest the wrong kinds of fats or not enough of the right kind, then that is when you will get high cholesterol levels. So do yourself a favor, keep it simple and eat the right kinds of fats, very easy and simple to follow. Leave the rest, don't buy the hype and erroneous myths. There is no need to worry about high cholesterol levels if you eat a balanced and natural diet for your body type. **Another funny myth exposed and vaporized!**

The Eat Lean Meats Myth

In recent years there has been a shift of people starting to eat leaner cuts of meat such as chicken breast, lean red meat portions and other meats of leaner type. It is proposed that eating leaner meats is healthier than eating fattier portions of meat as in chicken wings and chicken legs and rib eye steaks and ground beef. Well my friend, yep... you guessed it, just another funny myth being proposed as healthy. Let me simply provide basic holistic science facts and common sense because that is all you require to see the Truth. Eating lean cuts of meats actually promotes low levels of health and causes your body to become depleted of nutrients and creates an acidic environment internally. Lean meat is pure protein and requires extra enzymes and other bio-nutrients to break down the protein so that your body may make use of it to supply itself for nutrition.

Excessive consumption of lean meats causes all sorts of health disorders and places strain on the liver and colon. By the way, eating fatty portions of meat DOES NOT clog arteries as is being proposed. The clogged arteries come from other factors such as the consumption of unhealthy hydrogenated fats, excessive sugar intake which leads to yeast and parasite formation and other metabolic wastes in the body that accumulate. You may actually get artery clogging by ingesting excessive amounts of lean meats since the body becomes acidic and then requires buffering it out and thus form stones and calcium formations. Calcium is the main buffer mineral used by the body to neutralize acids and other harmful waste products. The more acidic your body becomes the more your body has to use reserve calcium to buffer these acids and eventually this excess calcium will turn into stones and other calcifications. Have you ever seen that white formation around water spigots and other water drains? That is calcium buildup and is the similar process going on when excess calcium is used to buffer the acids in your body. So in essence you are doing yourself a disservice by consuming lean portions of meats.

The Truth is that eating the fattier portions of meats as in chicken wings and legs and the inners of the chicken, rib eye steaks, ground beef (the fattier the better) and other fatty meats is absolutely healthy and promote good health. The main thing is to moderate your portions. A portion the size of your hand is a great guide to follow when eating meats. Also be sure to balance your meal with enough fresh veggies. In fact, my recommendation is to always have half of your plate be fresh steamed veggies. The main issue of today and why people are experiencing health disorders is that they have their portions and their meat options way off. They are eating big portions of lean meats, a large serving of starch food and a super small portion of vegetable. This causes acidity in the body which leads to numerous health disorders and places undue stress on your organs. The key is to alter the ratios and the meat options and then you are on the right track.

A healthy meal consists of fresh steamed veggies or raw, a complex starch food as in brown rice or wild rice, or whole grain spouted bread and then a small portion of fatty meat as in chicken legs or rib eye steak. This meal is balanced and has the proper ratio of fats to starches to protein. Also, another fact to become aware of is that eating fattier portions of meats is actually easier on your body. Fatty meat is easier to digest and requires less enzymes and bio-nutrients to break down. And...the secret that your body knows which is healthier...the lean or the fatty meat. This is so simple but again you have been programmed to go against what nature has intended. So, do yourself a simple experiment...or even just think about it in a common sense way...if you have 2 options before you, one is a plate of lean chicken breast and the other plate has 3 chicken legs...which does your body feel a pull toward? Which do you really want to eat? Which tastes better and feels better when you eat it? Pretty simple!

Another funny myth exposed and vaporized. Ah...Ba Buy!

Foundational Holistic Health Truths For Healthy Living

Digestion, Assimilation & Elimination

Proper digestion, assimilation and elimination are the absolute key factors of feeling and looking your best. Digestion of food and the assimilation of the nutrients in that food are the two most important components of your health. After your body has completed the process of digestion and assimilation, the left over bulk leaves your body via elimination through your colon. In an optimally healthy person this process works efficiently and effectively.

Your main intention when eating food should be: ingest foods that contain a balance of nutrients and have those nutrients get into your cells. However, when your body is polluted and you have a congested liver and colon due to impacted food substance, your digestion is weak and your assimilation of nutrients is poor leading to severe deficiencies.

When you are toxic internally, your body and cells cannot digest your food and convert that food into energy for your body. In fact, you are depleting your body of energy and your cells of nutrients when you do not have a clean internal cellular environment. So, instead of nourishing and energizing your body, you are taxing an already weak system. Thus, you may experience fatigue, tiredness, and overall poor health. For some people they may be only digesting and assimilating around 30% to 50% of the food they eat. This is due to a toxic intercellular environment, a congested liver and a poor elimination system from the colon being impacted with toxins and old food materials.

There really is only one key way to improve all aspects of digestion, assimilation and elimination of the food you ingest. Detoxification of your entire body is absolutely critical for improving all these components of your health. These processes will not improve unless you clean the cells and body of all toxicities and impurities that do not belong there. It is pointless to take supplements to remedy this condition. When your body is full of pollutants, it will not be able to assimilate all the compounds and nutrients in the supplement.

I recommend cleaning your body and cells appropriately before engaging in a supplemental program. You will save a lot of money and will receive more benefits from the foods and supplements you ingest when you are clean from the inside and have proper digestion, assimilation and elimination. You will learn more information on proper detoxification in a later chapter.

Helpful tips for better digestion and assimilation:

1) Chew your food well. Understand that your stomach does not have teeth and is not meant to break down food. Your stomach is simply a chamber where the appropriate acids and enzymes mix with the food you eat and creates the proper pH for that food to break down to be ready for the next phase of digestion. When you only chew your food a few times before swallowing you make the job of your stomach and the rest of your body much harder. This leads to mal-digestion and can stress your whole digestive system in general.

2) Only eat the proper kinds of foods together. I suggest eating only protein foods with vegetables or carbohydrate foods with vegetables only. Eating carbohydrate foods (bread, pasta) with protein foods (meat, cheese, eggs) can lead to mal-digestion and fatigue. Also do not eat sweet foods with main meals. This sets up fermentation in your system leading to mal-digestion, bad breath, body odor and overall poor health.

3) Take the proper digestive enzymes after all main meals. Supplementing with the proper enzymes will aid your digestion and assimilation of nutrients. The enzymes will help break down food and provide the proper pH levels for an efficient process.

A Strong Defense Against Illness

Maintaining a strong immune system is the key to living a life free from illness.

When your immune system is functioning at its peak performance, then illness simply cannot set it. It would be in your best interest to ensure that your immune system is always functioning optimally if you wish to avoid any health disorder. So, how do you ensure that your immune system is working at its best? The key to an optimally functioning immune system is by maintaining a high level of healthy bacteria (probiotics) in your digestive and intestinal tract. However, your immunity may not be functioning at peak performance due to environmental pollution, stress, and poor eating habits.

I would say that stress is the number one factor that contributes to poor immunity. Stress can cause havoc on your immune system by disrupting key biological processes needed for optimum health. Stress can leave your whole body in an unbalanced state. Due to the profound impact that stress can have on your body and immune system, this can leave you very susceptible to many health disorders. In fact, stress usually gets stored in the body and cells weakening organs, disrupting digestion, hormone regulation, cell communication, nutrient transport, and even impacts your mental and emotional health.

It is my recommendation to find an avenue to release stress as best you can on a regular basis. Massage therapy, yoga, meditation, sports, playing, and walking in nature are great ways to release stress from your body. Also, changing your perspective of life in general can work wonders to reduce stress. How do you change your perspective? Perhaps you could view life in a different context. View life as a game and not something where you go through the motions day in and day out. Picture it as a grand game or an exciting movie where you can choose to play any part you wish. Simply know that you can change parts/roles anytime you wish. Use your imagination and you will experience miracles.

Aside from reducing stress from your life, the best way to improve immunity is by consuming high quality probiotic supplements. Obviously, eating a well-balanced diet with fruits, vegetables, wholesome foods, essential fatty acids, enzymes, trace minerals and drinking plenty of purified Living Water will further ensure that your immune system works at its best. Consuming probiotics on a frequent basis is essential to obtaining and maintaining optimum health.

More than seventy percent of your immune system is centered in and around the digestive and intestinal tract. You may not know this important fact. It is interesting that the majority of your defense system that protects you from illness is little bacteria. These live bacteria have a host of other functions beyond protecting your body from illness. They are responsible for aiding in digestion, assimilating nutrients, transporting nutrients, exterminating parasites, fungi, candida, viruses, and clean your intestinal membranes of toxins and other harmful compounds. Live bacteria also ensure that you eliminate properly

Elimination is paramount to health. If you are not eliminating your waste every day, then you can be sure you have serious deficiencies in not only live bacteria (probiotics) but also nutrients. Bowel elimination is critical for keeping a clean body. If you eliminate frequently then you have a good digestion and a healthy immune system. If you eliminate infrequently, then this is a sign that your immunity and overall health may be poor regardless of how you feel.

Infrequent bowel movements also signifies that you are toxic, meaning that your body is accumulating harmful compounds since they are not being excreted in a normal fashion through your waste. Keep in mind that health disorders take time to build up. You may feel pretty good now but deep in your body are conditions that may be unfavorable to long term health.

It is essential to consume the right kind of probiotics. There are many products available in the market place. Most of these products do not contain enough live organisms to be of significant benefit to your body. Some products contain other ingredients such as fillers, binders, and delivery support compounds. It is important to know what to look for in a high quality probiotic supplement. I recommend liquid probiotic products over the capsule versions for numerous reasons.

A good probiotic supplement will contain a high amount of live organisms numbering in the billions. Also, no fillers or binders should be present. Live bacteria need food to survive. A good probiotic supplement should contain a food source for the live bacteria to feed on to ensure the organisms survive for a period of time after product manufacturing is complete. Also, you need to make sure that the bacteria strains survive digestive and stomach acids when you ingest them. I recommend taking live coconut kefir drinks as they seem to be the most potent and viable.

Maintaining a high level of vital bacteria in your body is one of the most important practices that you can follow. I recommend starting a program of incorporating probiotics into your daily diet immediately. Consuming probiotics with meals is best since the food will aid in feeding these little guys while traveling down your digestive and intestinal tract.

The Sugar Blues

It would be fair to assume that almost everyone on the planet loves sugar and sweet foods. Processed sugar is in many products and is a key ingredient for baking. It seems that everyone has a sweet tooth for sugar food in one way or another. Most people know to limit their intake of processed sugar; however, what you may not know is that sugar is one of the worst ingredients that you can put into your body. The chemical reaction of sugar in the body acts as a poison. Actually, studies show that sugar has drug like effects in the body.

Processed sugar has many harmful effects throughout the body and can cause major imbalances in the organ systems. You could say that sugar tends to throw off the homeostatic balance of the whole body by increasing the production of adrenaline. In essence, sugar stimulates the nervous system by inducing a flight or fight response. This is obviously not a healthy process. This intense reaction of the body increases the production of cortisone, which suppresses immune function and can lead to other health disorders.

The daily intake of sugar leads to many other imbalances and malfunctioning of the bodily processes. High sugar consumption typically leads to an overly acidic body and in turn will cause the body to strip nutrients from its reserves to counterbalance this effect. This can eventually cause the body to take calcium from the bones and teeth since calcium is the primary mineral used to neutralize high acid in the cells. Osteoporosis and arthritic conditions can result from this continued process.

Sugar and its Link to Weight Gain

Excess sugar consumption will eventually affect every organ in the body. Primarily, sugar is stored in the liver as glucose. Since the liver's capacity to store sugar in this form is limited, the liver will start to expand almost like a balloon with continued daily sugar intake. When the livers' capacity has been filled, the excess glycogen (glucose) is returned to the blood in the form of fatty acids (fat). The fatty acid compounds are then taken to various parts of the body and are stored as fat deposits in the buttocks, belly, breasts and hips since these are the most inactive body parts.

The consumption of excess processed (refined) carbohydrates has the same effect on the body. Eating foods with refined white flours and other enriched products can cause the same physiological effects. Consuming excess pasta, rice, chips, pretzels, and other high processed carbohydrates can lead to fat deposits on the body. Many people do not understand how eating excess pasta or rice can cause weight gain since these foods have very minute quantities of fat and low calories in them. The secret: it's not that important how much fat or calories a food has. The real key is what biological effect a food has once in the body.

When the inactive body parts have become filled with fat then eventually the excess fatty acid deposits will become stored around major organ systems such as the heart and kidneys. This leads to the degeneration of these organs and, in turn, poor health. This can result in poor immune response, poor circulation, high blood pressure, and can even impact brain functioning.

A False Energy High

Too much sugar intake gives you a false sense of energy. When you eat a sweet food, your energy will go up; however, it only feels that your energy is going up. In fact, this false energy is really your body being stimulated via the flight or fight response that I spoke of earlier. After this reaction has worn off, your energy levels will come crashing down as most people experience every day after they have eaten a high sugar food.

Most children that have ADD and/or ADHD can usually heal themselves simply by eliminating processed sugars in their diets. Children typically eat way too many processed sugars. The behaviors and bodily responses that these children feel are often the flight or fight responses of their nervous systems.

All forms of processed sugars such as Nutra Sweet, cane juice, corn syrup, brown sugar, Splenda, powdered sugar and others have the same effect on the body. The chemical structures of these compounds are very harmful to the body and should not be consumed on a frequent basis.

Fruit sugars are very healthy for you. The monosaccharaides (simple sugars) in these natural foods are in a structure that is beneficial to your cells. Fruit sugar has a much different effect on your body than does processed sugar. Fruit sugars nourish and energize the body naturally. This is true energy as compared to the false energy one gets from processed sugars. Your cells require the simple sugars in fruits consistently since they serve to fuel the body with the best substances. Make sure you consistently eat many fruits a day. I recommend eating 2 pieces of different fruits a day for better health.

The True Bitterness of Nutra Sweet & Splenda (sucralose).

Aspartame (Nutra Sweet) is actually worse to consume than sugar. This technical name includes the following brands of sweeteners- (Equal, Nutra Sweet, Spoonful and Equal Measure).

Be advised that these compounds are very powerful and can cause severe biological effects in your body. To say that they are toxic is an understatement.

The Breakdown of Aspartame In Your Body

Aspartame is a volatile substance, meaning that it breaks down very readily under normal storing conditions. Primarily, once ingested all aspartame compounds break down into methanol (alcohol), which is a known neurotoxin. The methanol in time will break down into formaldehyde, a highly reactive chemical that is damaging to the cells and genetics of the body. This process can cause a number of neurodegenerative diseases such as Alzheimer's, lupus, multiple sclerosis (MS), and Parkinson's disease. The methyl alcohol that forms from aspartame is thousands of times more potent than the alcohol found in a normal alcoholic beverage.

Reactions to aspartame products include the following: headaches, nausea, depression, fatigue, heart palpitations, slurred speech, breathing difficulties, memory loss, seizures. Consuming high amounts of aspartame can also increase your cravings for carbohydrates. Primarily, the effects of aspartame chemicals in the body seem to alter key hormones thus creating imbalances in neurotransmitters and blocking other hormone precursors.

Aspartame & Children

Children love to consume sweets on a daily basis. Many of the food products these children are consuming have aspartame sweeteners in them. I would advise all parents to get their kids off of aspartame food items. These foods are not healthy for them. There are plenty of healthy alternatives for any of the items.

Many kids are diagnosed with ADD and other mood disorders. Many of these conditions are being classified as hyper, behavioral problems and others when in fact these children are being affected by the foods they eat. Look at a normal child's food intake for an average day and you will find that they eat way too much sugar and items with aspartame compounds in them. This daily consumption of these sweeteners has a harmful effect on their nervous system and therefore becomes expressed as mood disorders and behavioral problems. Take these kids off sugar and sweeteners and watch them improve.

Pregnant Mothers & Aspartame

If you or anyone you know is pregnant then I would highly recommend staying away from these dangerous sweeteners forever. Make sure you read labels and make it a conscious intent to have the whole family keep clean of these products. It will help your whole family out I assure you. If you are pregnant and consume aspartame foods you will only be hurting the development of the child. Doing so can cause neurological imbalances and other cellular damage. You are also hurting yourself. It is not worth the price to have your diet soda. Please educate yourself more on this topic for it can save your health and the baby's health.

Products to Stay Away From

If you drink diet soda then are you most likely consuming aspartame. Most diet sodas and many other beverages are sweetened with one of the aspartame sugar substitutes. STAY AWAY FROM ALL PRODUCTS THAT CONTAIN THE VARIOUS FORMS OF ASPARTAME! These include aspartame, Nutra Sweet, Splenda, Spoonful, Equal. Read your labels and throw away all items that have these compounds in them. Take responsibility for your diet. If you choose to continue to consume aspartame after reading this chapter, well, then you are the one to pay the consequences.

What Can You Use To Sweeten Drinks & My Food

Relax! I know you enjoy sugar and do not want to give up great tasting foods and beverages. You don't have to. There are some great natural sugar alternatives that I feel taste better than sugar and the other toxic substances mentioned earlier. To sweeten your drinks you can use banana put into a magic bullet with your drink.

Raw Honey is a great food product to use as a sweetener. Organic maple syrup is also a good sugar alternative. It can be used in various ways and has a pleasant taste. Yacon syrup is also a very nutritive food that can be used to sweeten drinks and baked goods, even pancakes. Give it try. Banana puree can also be used for baking. Great stuff!

I would recommend buying some of these sweeteners and see which ones you like. They are all fairly healthy to consume on regular basis and you will feel the difference. You will not miss regular sugar, believe me. Your body will thank you!

The Shadow Side of Soy

The products that have emerged into the market that are made from soy are numerous. In many stores across the country you see shelves stocked with products made from this legume. There is extensive information and profound claims that soy is very healthy to one's health. There are claims from being able to lower cholesterol to even fighting cancer.

The bounty of information is endless that promotes soy as a miracle food. Many doctors and nutritionists recommend including soy as a part of the diet for the health benefits. People of all ages seem to be accepting of this product in various forms. You may be using this product yourself in the hopes of receiving the health benefits. So, soy is healthy huh…Oh really now?

Contrary to what most people have been led to believe, soy can actually be quite harmful to your health if eaten frequently. What many researchers aren't revealing is that soybeans contain large quantities of natural toxins or anti-nutrients.

The first category of anti-nutrient found in soybeans are enzyme inhibitors that block the action of trypsin, an anti-cancer enzyme, and other enzymes that are needed to digest proteins properly. These compounds aren't deactivated during cooking. These toxins can cause serious gastric distress and reduced protein digestion in the body. They can also increase your chances of getting cancer. Soybeans also contain compounds called haemaglutinins, a clot promoting substance. These can actually cause the red blood cells to clump together. They can also serve as a growth depressant causing abnormal development in humans. Another harmful compound found in soybeans is goitrogens, which can actually depress thyroid function.

In recent years, there have been studies to show that soy consumption is not really healthy as claimed. Soybeans are also high in phytic acid that can serve to block the uptake of essential minerals in the intestinal tract. When there is a high phytic acid level in the diet, essential minerals like calcium, magnesium, copper, iron and especially zinc cannot be absorbed properly by the body. This is obviously not a healthy situation since these minerals are vital for optimum health. Vegetarians who eat soy as their main source of protein are doing themselves a great disservice since they are risking becoming deficient in these essential minerals.

Zinc is especially important for optimal development and functioning of the brain and nervous system. Zinc is also responsible for a healthy immune system and blood sugar control. I would advise vegetarians to gradually wean themselves off soy based foods and incorporate more beans and whole grains like Kamut, Spelt, Millet, Quinoa, and Oats into their diets. These grains contain high amounts of protein and are healthy to consume on a frequent basis. Sprouted versions of these grains are the best option since they are better digested and assimilated by the cells.

Soy & Infants

Around 25% of bottle fed children in this country receive a soy-based formula as their main source of nutrition. There are many pediatricians that recommend soy based formulas if an infant does not do well with regular milk formulas. Well, there are scientists that have known for years that feeding children soy formula can cause thyroid problems. Soy infant feeding can also be the cause of many other health disorders in children such as diabetes and hormonal irregularities.

Thyroid disease is very common among children who consume a soy- based formula since the isoflavones found in this product can depress the thyroid and cause it to malfunction. Isoflavones are estrogen like substances, which can have the same effect as the body's estrogen. Too much estrogen in the body can result in serious disorders. There are many reported stories from parents regarding the feeding of soy formula to their children. They range from emotional behavior problems, asthma, immune disorders, irritable bowel syndrome, thyroid disorder, and even abnormal development.

Healthy Soy

There are certain forms of soy that can be healthy for you. These would include anything that is made from either fermented soy or sprouted soy. These food products are items like miso, tempeh, and other food items that contain fermented or sprouted soy. These forms of soy can supply you with health benefits. In fact, the Asian cultures eat primarily these fermented and sprouted forms of soy. This is where the west got all of its information about the health benefits of soybeans.

If you consume soy on a regular basis, I would advise that you reduce your intake to a minimal level or find a new substitute to consume. Eating soy once a week will probably not hurt you but if you consume soy several times a week then you could subject yourself to future harm. Please take time to educate yourself a little more on this topic. After having all of the facts you will see that it will be easy to make the healthiest choice possible for your wellbeing.

Cayenne Pepper, The Master Healer

Cayenne pepper is known to some as one of the greatest all natural remedies.

Many refer to this divine substance as a cure-all. It has many properties that can facilitate healing for many ailments. Most people know Cayenne pepper as a spice to add to their food. However, there are many hidden healing properties within this compound. It is one of the best sources of vitamin C and has very powerful anti-oxidants. The vitamins within this substance can destroy harmful bacteria in the body. It also serves as a major antiseptic formula for the cells. Cayenne pepper is known to contain certain flavonoids that can help people with heart conditions by healing unhealthy heart cells. It can also increase blood circulation throughout the body immediately upon ingestion.

Cayenne can also work to remove deposits throughout the body where there is stagnation of certain organs. Anyone who has ever ingested this compound knows of the immediate physiological and metabolic effects it has. This is what makes this divine substance so profound. You don't have to wait for the body to process it. In fact, there are biochemical changes that occur as soon as it is placed in your mouth. Talk about efficient!

Cayenne pepper is used by certain cultures for the known healing effects. Some cultures use it as a digestion aid because it contains enzymes that helps the body break down food more efficiently and helps the stomach secrete more acids. Other known therapies used are for the treatment and removal of parasites and other harmful bacteria that can house themselves in the body.

In fact, Cayenne pepper has the ability to boost immunity dramatically. In times when someone is sick with a cold or flu, they can decrease the severity and longevity of their symptoms significantly. Sinus congestion can be greatly reduced and sore throat eliminated much faster if one consumes Cayenne during their sickness period.

The following is a remedy you can use in times of a cold or flu:

- Brew a big pot of caffeine free tea: chamomile, peppermint, Echinacea, etc.

- Place a big pinch of ORGANIC Cayenne pepper in AFTER it has cooled to room temperature. Heating destroys the active compounds that are healing.

- Add a small piece of ginger mashed up as well.

- Teaspoon of raw honey .Sip this throughout the day and notice how you feel.

Cayenne pepper also has the ability to make all other nutrients and supplements you take more effective by increasing the function of the body to absorb these substances. Many compounds that are taken by people to target certain ailments never get to the area that it is intended for because their circulation is not functioning properly. However, when you take Cayenne pepper with another substance, it dramatically improves the circulation of the whole body ensuring that it gets to the area of interest.

For example, let's say someone is taking glucosamine for his or her joints or arthritis. Many times this compound will not reach the joints as intended due to poor circulation and therefore will get eliminated from the body. If we were able to increase the circulation of this person and then have them take the glucosamine, you would find that now the substance would be better absorbed by the body and work as intended to restore joint health.

Cayenne pepper can also be used as a remedy to stop bleeding. In fact, it works so well that it can stop most bleeding and injuries within minutes. There are clotting properties contained within this compound. These clotting properties work to constrict blood vessels so that bleeding stops immediately upon contact. If you ever experience a cut, wash it immediately with running water. Next, place Cayenne powder directly onto the wound. This will serve to not only stop the bleeding but also sterilizes and keeps it from acquiring additional bacteria and germs.

This is a good remedy product to carry if you have kids since they are always playing and getting scraped or cut. Place a small vial or bottle of Cayenne in your handbag. In emergencies simply place a small pinch on the wound. Wrap the wound afterwards with a gauze or band-aid. You can also add a little honey to the wound the day after since the honey will nourish the cells and keep the wound protected from bacteria or germs that may cause infection. In fact, cuts or injuries that have Cayenne placed on them heal much faster than other traditional treatments.

Another remedy for Cayenne pepper is that it can be used for sore muscles, strains, sprains, swelling and inflammation. Simply make a rub out of it by placing a few teaspoons of Cayenne in some olive oil, almond oil, grapeseed oil or jojoba oil. Mix this and rub it real well right into the area of pain. Afterwards, take a hot towel and cover the area for 30 minutes. Do this repetitively for a number of days.

Cayenne contains high amounts of vitamin C and causes immediate physiological changes in your blood. It will give you an immediate surge of energy when taken orally. If you are ever feeling fatigued or drained simply place a few Cayenne grains on your tongue or put a pinch of Cayenne in juice and sip it. You will feel an immediate boost of energy since this compound doesn't need to be processed by the body. It goes directly into your bloodstream causing rapid physiological changes. Try it and you will see.

Cayenne is also known to eliminate headaches and migraines within minutes. Simply add a pinch to some water, tea or juice and drink this mixture when you feel a headache coming on. You will be amazed at the results! There are some important points to understand when using Cayenne as a remedy for health and healing. There are many forms and sources of Cayenne pepper available in the world. The more pure the ingredient is, the more powerful the effects are.

I would recommend buying organic ingredients only since these products do not contain pesticides and other harmful substances in them that could impact effectiveness. Also, if you have never taken Cayenne orally and would like to try this compound, please start off slowly. Use only a few grains at a time or place just a small pinch in some water or juice to allow your body to adjust to this very create better health.

Microwave Ovens - The Truth Revealed

Millions of people use microwave ovens because they are so convenient in preparing foods and beverages. Most people tend to think that these ovens are relatively safe to use. I mean, come on, millions of people use them so why wouldn't they be safe.

These scientific discoveries clearly show that the continued use of these appliances for food preparation has a harmful effect on the human body. In fact, the Russians have known about these dangers for decades and have outlawed microwave use in their country since the 1970's. Other European countries have found the same evidence, that microwaving foods in not healthy for the human body.

Essentially, microwaves use radiation energy to cook food. Radiation energy has been proven to be harmful to all living things. To apply this mode of cooking to our food is not beneficial to our health as common sense would tell anyone. However, misinformation and propaganda has programmed people to believe that microwave ovens are safe. Once again we have something that is common sense and yet millions of people do not see the truth right under their nose. This is how programming works. Time for some de-programming wouldn't you say?

How Microwave Ovens Work

Microwave ovens use short radiation waves to bombard the molecules of food, which creates friction among these molecules and causes the food to heat up. What isn't being revealed is that these radiation waves rip the food molecules apart deforming them. What does this mean? It means that micro-waved food is molecularly altered. It no longer carries the natural biological makeup for that specific food. This change in the food molecules creates foreign and toxic substances. When you ingest these altered compounds, they can disrupt natural bodily processes and affect your health. It has been scientifically observed that amino acids in micro-waved food have been transformed into unhealthy compounds. Also, studies have found that people consuming food cooked in microwave ovens had significant changes in their blood.

Dr. Hans Ulrich Hertel, a Lausanne University professor (Swiss) published a research paper on his study of microwave ovens and their harmful effects on food and people. The scientific conclusion showed that using a microwave oven to cook with, molecularly altered the nutrients in food. More importantly, his findings showed changes in the blood of the participants of the study that were conducive to degeneration and breakdown.

The following are some of the findings of Russian investigations into the use of microwave ovens:

- Microwaving meats caused the production of d- Nitrosodienthanolamines, which are known to be carcinogenic.

- Microwaving milk and cereals caused their amino acids to be transformed into carcinogenic compounds.

- Microwaving raw or frozen vegetables caused the plant alkaloids to be converted to carcinogenic compounds.

- The nutrients of all micro-waved foods were substantially altered.

- Decreased availability of vitamins and minerals of all tested foods

Microwave Ovens and Heating Baby's Milk

People who have had a baby typically use a microwave oven to heat their baby's milk. PARENTS BEWARE!! Heating the bottle in a microwave oven can cause changes in the milk, primarily destroying minerals and changes in other properties of the milk. Studies have shown that heating baby formula in microwave ovens can alter the amino acids and form carcinogens.

Many parents use baby formula instead of nursing their baby naturally. This baby formula is not healthy to begin with. Combine this unhealthy baby formula with heating in a microwave oven and now you have a real dangerous concoction. I would advise all parents not to heat baby milk (formula) in microwave ovens. Use warm water under the sink or simply heat some water in a pot and then put the bottle into the pot. Make sure it is not too hot. Test it on your hand first. This is a good indicator.

What You Can Do To Heat Up Your Foods

Why do you need to use a microwave oven? Answer that question! You use it because you have been conditioned to think it is harmless and because it is convenient. Do you want to eat molecularly altered (TOXIC) food? Or do you want to eat food that is in its natural form? It is about choices.

Suggestions:

With thawing meat, get a large bowl and put hot water into it. Put your meat in and leave for 10 minutes. Add more hot water after 10 minutes or until thawed. You can thaw meat in just about the same time it takes in a microwave using this method. Use this method for thawing vegetables too.

Use a toaster oven to thaw breads or other baked goods. Use your imagination and you will be just fine without a microwave oven, believe me. If you value your health then you will get rid of your microwave oven as soon as possible. Don't give it away, just go down to your local junkyard and see if they will buy it from you for scrap metal. If not, LEAVE AT THE JUNK YARD!

If you are thinking of using your microwave oven to heat up water for tea, coffee or any other beverage, THINK AGAIN! The radiation waves have the same effect on the molecules of water. In fact, water is much more easily altered when heated in a microwave oven. Do not heat water in a microwave oven! You are setting yourself up for harm. GET RID OF THE THING!!

The Flu Shot Deception

Every year around November many people go and receive the flu shot in the hopes of avoiding getting sick. Many people believe that by getting a flu shot they will reduce their chances of becoming sick with that year's strain of flu virus. The media reminds everyone at the onset of fall to go and receive their yearly shot. At times it is stated on the news that there may not be enough flu shots to supply everyone who wants one.

Does this once a year shot actually reduce your chances of getting the flu? Well, where do I begin? I will use simple science to show that the flu shot cannot work as is claimed and is a MAJOR SCAM!!!

Science Fact or Science Fiction? You decide.

First of all, the flu virus mutates every year. In essence, the flu virus has a different biological makeup every single year. Until the flu virus mutates no one in the world can possibly know the new mutated biological makeup of it. However, doctors and scientists claim that they can predict what the new biological makeup of the flu virus will be in advance. From this prediction, they produce a serum, which is then used for that year's flu shot solution.

No one except the grand CREATOR of the universe can possibly know what the new virus will look like before it actually mutates. It is almost like saying that you can predict what the weather will be like exactly on a specific date many months in advance. I don't think so! Learn to discern what you hear on the news about health. It is of critical importance that you begin to question what you are hearing on TV or hearing on the radio.

Another interesting fact about the flu shot is that by receiving a dose of it, you have actually increased your chances of getting flu-like symptoms. How? Well, by receiving a flu shot, you now have injected a flu virus into your body. You now may experience flu- like symptoms because your immune system will try to eliminate the injected virus. This is a normal physiological response to any virus that enters the body.

It makes no sense whatsoever to inject a virus into your body when you are trying to avoid getting this virus in the first place. Can you see the irony here?? A major fact worth noting is that at least fifty percent of people who receive the flu shot end up getting the flu anyway. If you think about what I have just disclosed to you about the deception of the flu shot you will see how true my words are. It doesn't take a rocket scientist to put the pieces together.

Only the creator of this vast universe knows the future strain of any virus. Empower yourself and learn truth! It is always there waiting to be discovered. It is up to you to go discover it!

Thus, the claims in favor of the flu shot are preposterous to say the least. You actually have less of a chance of getting the flu simply by not getting a flu shot. Also, you can further reduce your chances significantly by taking a few precautionary measures.

Here's a fact for you: More than 50% of the people who get the flu shot end up getting the flu or flu-like symptoms.

You can significantly reduce your chances of getting the flu by incorporating some very simple habits into your daily regimen. Here is secret that you may not know...simply because you get exposed to the flu virus does not mean that you will get the flu.

Here are 10 simple ways to reduce your chances of getting the flu every year:

1) Wash your hands with essential oil soap frequently throughout the day.

2) Drink about 2 liters of high quality structured water per day.

3) Spray ionized super silver in your ears, eyes and nose before you leave your house in the morning and a few times throughout the day in the fall and winter

months.

4) Reduce you stress levels. Stress has the biggest impact on your immune system is the #1 reason why people fall ill with the flu.

5) Eat a highly balanced diet consisting of fruits and vegetables, healthy fats and protein.

6) Take 1 tablespoon of Fish oil or Hemp Seed several times a week.

7) Make sure you are taking a good green powder and electrolyte supplement.

8) Take Echinacea and elderberry tincture or tea 3 to 5 times per week in the fall and winter.

9) Make sure you are getting some sun exposure every day as this will help your body create vitamin D which is critical for health and warding off illness.

10) Rub 2 drops of essential oil like lavender, eucalyptus, peppermint or lemon into your wrist area every morning in the fall and winter months.

Juicing green veggies can also be a healthy practice in the winter months. Organic Cayenne pepper in tea is also very good to take in the winter months to ward off any type of colds and flu.

If you do come down with a cold or flu, then it is best not to take any over the counter products. These products have numerous chemicals in them. The last thing you want to do is add chemicals into your body when you are sick. This is not wise. When your body is sick, it requires natural compounds.

Here are some great tips for reducing the symptoms of the cold and flu:

Upon noticing symptoms, immediately take a homeopathic flu remedy as prescribed.

1) Take a high quality probiotic liquid product every two to three hours.

2) Take a high quality Echinacea supplement and be sure to spray your ears and nose with ionic silver every few hours throughout the day.

3) Add 1 tablespoon of fresh ginger to organic chamomile tea. Brew a big pot of this tea and sip this all day long while adding fresh ginger to each cup you drink. This will reduce many of your symptoms.

4)   Another excellent natural remedy for knocking out the flu or cold faster is to swab your ear canals and nostrils with cotton swabs that are saturated with nano-silver or ionic silver. Do this every 2 to 3 hours around the clock. This is very effective and can dramatically help to reduce symptoms.

5) Drink lots of structured water throughout the day to flush out toxins.

6) Eat only light foods like soups and broths, steamed vegetables, and healthy oils like hemp seed, coconut oil and fish oils. Stay away from dairy since these foods cause phlegm and mucus to form.

7) Take a hot bath with sea salts, Magnesium and essential oils like peppermint or eucalyptus.

Germs Can't Hurt You

If you are healthy and follow a comprehensive health regimen then viruses or bacteria can not affect you. You see, the germ theory that has been propagated over the years since Lou Pasteur has been debunked. Even Pasteur himself said before he passed that his theory was flawed and he felt that germs did play a role in illness and poor health; however, they are not the root cause for any illness. The grand truth is that you can significantly reduce your chances of getting the flu. How? Well, your emotional and mental state will have more to do with you getting the flu than being exposed to the virus itself. Simply because you may be exposed to the flu virus, does not mean that you will get sick. People come in contact with bacteria and many viruses every single day of their lives.

If it were as simple as being exposed to a virus to become sick, then we would all be sick every day of our lives. It doesn't work that way! You become sick when you are not balanced in mind, body, and spirit. When you have emotional distress, mental stress, stress from everyday life and then you couple this with not eating properly and/or sleeping adequately, this sets you up for becoming sick.

Vaccines and Their Dangers

A major point worth noting is that vaccines do not prevent illness.
Vaccines were initially developed on the primary basis of a theory. It was
theorized that vaccines would work as claimed. The evidence clearly shows that
they do not work as intended.

In fact, vaccines contain many carcinogenic compounds in them such as
thimerosol, a mercury derivative, formaldehyde, and other harmful ingredients.
Many people have been harmed by these toxic compounds, especially small
children. These harmful compounds can overwhelm a child's immune system
and cause severe conditions such as autism and other autoimmune disorders.

Another interesting fact is that vaccines are not responsible for the decline
in some of the past epidemics. People have been led to believe that the
vaccination program has been responsible for the eradication for certain
diseases. The decline in these diseases can be attributed to the advancements in
technologies and higher standards of living throughout the world.

Many of the epidemics from the past can be attributed to poor living
standards and malnutrition. When you have thousands of people living in close
proximity of each other and there are no septic systems in place, this is where
the seed for epidemics can flourish. As the case many years ago, there were
many people living in small towns with no sewage treatment plants. This means

that many of these people were coming in contact with other people's bodily fluids.

Whenever you come in contact with another person's fecal matter or other bodily fluids, you set yourself up for many illnesses. This was the main cause of all past epidemics. In fact, this is a major health problem still in India and other third world nations today. In India for example, there are millions of people living in major cities that have no sewage treatment plants whatsoever. In essence, you have many people's bodily fluids all over the place. This is a perfect breeding ground for epidemics and in fact India has many epidemics running rampant still today because many of the cities have no sewage treatment systems.

So, the decline in certain diseases in the United States is not a result of the vaccination program. The decline is directly a result of better living conditions and better health standards in general. Sewage treatment plants have been a major reason for the decline in many of the epidemics. Better nutrition and healthier living environments are also a major reason for the eradication of many diseases. In fact, many of the past epidemics were already on the decline even before the vaccination program began.

I will close in saying that there is more than enough proof to validate what I am saying. I would say do your own research and see for yourself.

I would recommend educating yourself so that you can be empowered with knowledge to protect yourself from unneeded harm. Do the research because you owe it to yourself and your family to know of things that could potentially hurt you or someone you love. What you don't know can hurt you!

To Salt or Not to Salt?

Salt is used extensively to flavor the foods we eat. We know that salt is needed by our bodies to function properly. Even animals require this substance to maintain proper health. So, why is it that doctors recommend reducing sodium consumption from your diet? Supposedly, excess salt consumption can lead to high blood pressure and other health conditions. Some patients like diabetics are placed on salt–free diets as to avoid other health issues. So, should we consume salt or should we not?

The true fact of the matter is that ordinary table salt is not a healthy substance to consume. There are many factors as to why this is so. First and most important is that table salt has been altered from its original composition. Ordinary table salt is typically heated to high temperatures and has been treated with chemicals. When mined salt is heated to high temperatures, the chemical structure is altered and is thus no longer true salt. The sodium chloride molecular structure is in essence converted into the molecular structure of sodium hydroxate. This chemical structure is quite harmful to your cells.

Also, aluminum silicate is added to table salt to make it free flowing. Aluminum is a very toxic compound. It is no wonder that doctors recommend reducing salt consumption. They simply don't know why salt is harmful in large quantities. Sodium is a needed substance for proper bodily function. If ordinary table salt is unhealthy, then how can you receive the sodium that is required for your body to function properly? There is really only one form of true sodium that the body can use and that is ORGANIC SODIUM. Organic sodium is a compound found in most fruits, vegetables and sea plants. This is the only true sodium compound that the cells of your body need in order to function properly.

Sodium has many functions in the body. It is a very important mineral and has a dramatic impact on your overall health. The following are just a few of the functions of sodium. A major function of sodium is to regulate overall water content of the cells. Without a proper balance of water inside and outside the cell, the body cannot function in an optimum state. Sodium is also responsible for overall energy production of the cells. Many times when people feel fatigued, they are really low on their sodium levels. Healthy bone formation requires optimum levels of sodium in the cells. Osteoporosis often times is attributed to not only having low calcium levels but also very low organic sodium levels in the body.

A misconception that exists about sodium is that high salt consumption results in high blood pressure. This is only true for the consumption of ordinary table salt. Table salt raises blood pressure because it is toxic and creates an unhealthy cellular environment. True organic sodium DOES NOT raise blood pressure and in fact regulates it for better health. Other functions of sodium are for a healthy libido, nerve cell communication, food absorption, regulating and balancing blood sugar levels.

There is one alternative to table salt that is very healthy to consume. The substance that I am referring to is SEA SALT. Sea salt is a very healthy additive for food and your health. Sea salt contains up to 80 trace minerals and is a pure compound. There are no chemicals added and no heating. It is pure salt that comes from seawater that has evaporated and left the residual compounds. Sea salt typically is gray in appearance and is sticky because it retains its moisture from the sea. In fact, sea salt has a better flavor than table salt. Table salt tends to have a metallic after taste. This is due to the aluminum added to it. Sea salt has a pure natural taste. You will taste the difference once you use it.

The 3 brands that I would recommend are Himalayan, Celtic and Real Salt. These are wonderful salts that can be purchased from most health food stores. You need to be careful when buying sea salt at the store. There are many other types of sea salt out at the market. The package may say sea salt on the label, however, it does not mean that it is pure.

How can you tell if the sea salt you have in front of you is pure? Look for the sea salt to be slightly gray in color and moist. There are some brands that are white in color like French Atlantic that are good. Also, look for the particle size to be somewhat course as compared to table salt. Read the label, it should say 100% Unrefined Sea Salt.

I find that the Himalayan sea salt is the best quality out on the market. Celtic sea salt would run second in my book. There are some other types of sea salt from other countries such as Australia and Europe. These can be good selections too.

You can use sea salt in baths as a stress reducer and a toxin remover for the body. You can use it as a facial scrubber and an exfoliator. You may also notice major improvements in your health once you start consuming sea salt on a regular basis. You may feel many wonderful things happening to your body. So sea salt it up because this stuff is great!

If you open your mind, you will see many truths that were once hidden.

Heartburn De-Gassed

Heartburn afflicts many people. Supposedly, as is claimed by western medicine, heartburn stems primarily from excess acid in the stomach. According to health officials, this excess acid is responsible for the chest pain and burning sensation one feels in their esophagus and chest area. It is claimed that by taking ant-acids, this excess acidity in the stomach and esophagus will be neutralized. There are now many advanced heartburn medications that are available to supposedly alleviate this condition. These heartburn products are intended to neutralize the excess acids.

The truth of the matter is that all of these heartburn claims are totally false. Heartburn is not directly due to excess acid in the stomach. Heartburn is directly attributed to a lack of acid and a lack of digestive enzymes in the stomach. Due to a lack of HCL and digestive enzymes, improper digestion occurs. Thus, food sits in the stomach longer than normal in which it ferments and putrefies or simply stated…IT ROTS! This results in the production of fermentation acids in the system. These acids can be quite potent. The burning sensation one feels in their chest and throat is due to the fact that this fermentation acid at times comes back up the esophagus.

A lack of acid and a lack of key digestive enzymes cause improper digestion, bloating, gas, and other symptoms attributed to heartburn. Common factors that are directly responsible for heartburn are; consumption of too many cooked (dead) foods, enzyme deficiency, dehydration, inadequate sodium levels, improper diet, essential fatty acid deficiency and stress. If you do not consume an adequate amount of water each day then you are dehydrated. Dehydration can lead to a production of less HCL (Hydrochloric acid). Aging can also be responsible for heartburn. As people age, the production of enzymes and normal bodily acids decrease. Improper diet is a very common factor for heartburn since most people in this country eat too many acidic foods.

Eating too many acidic foods can over time suppress the parietal cells in the stomach which are responsible for secreting Hydrochloric acid. Hydrochloric acid is mainly responsible for lowering stomach pH so that the proper enzymes can work to break down the food you eat. Foods such as pizza, hotdogs, french fries, meats, coffee, soda and other processed foods can do a number on your digestive system. By consuming these foods on a frequent basis, the parietal cells can become dysfunctional resulting in many digestive disorders. Also, you are depleting your body of enzymes when you eat dead (cooked) foods. This is why heartburn is so common.

The biggest mistake in attempting to alleviate heartburn is to take ant-acids. Even though these products may help you to feel better in the short run, they will only worsen your heartburn condition. By taking these products on a regular basis, you will further suppress any HCL acid that your body was producing. You see, ant-acids block or neutralize acids. As I have already stated, heartburn is really due to a lack of acid (HCL) in the stomach and a deficiency in key digestive enzymes. If you take a compound that blocks acids then you are actually worsening your heartburn condition because then the proper pH cannot be established in the stomach for enzymes to do their work.

Also, taking ant-acids long term interferes with digestion causing mal-absorption and eventually malnutrition. Ant-acids can also create an overly alkaline environment in the body. When you have an excess alkaline body environment, you set up a condition where calcium cannot be utilized by the cells. When your body is not absorbing calcium, you eventually reach a state of osteoporosis. Some ant-acid companies put calcium in their products. This is pointless since synthetic forms of calcium are not usable to your cells.

True Heartburn Relief

So, what can you do to rectify this condition? The first and most important step you can take is to restructure your diet. I would start with consuming more structured water and reach a level where you are drinking at least 2 to 3 liters a day (You can visit my website to discover how to create structured water for better hydration **MyBodyBrilliance.com**). Then, you can work on changing some of the foods you eat. Eating more raw and steamed vegetables will help tremendously since they contain many natural enzymes and minerals that will aid with digestion.

Eating fruit obviously is a major plus; however, I would recommend eating at least 1 piece a day. This practice will also help with supplying your cells with additional enzymes and will aid your body to function better overall. Papaya has many beneficial enzymes that will help you with digesting food properly. Another remedy is to sprinkle any or a combination of the following: cumin seeds, fennel seeds, pomegranate seeds, dry ginger, cardamom and tamarind bark on your foods. These spices contain many beneficial substances in them that will aid with digesting your food.

Reducing or eliminating some of the foods you eat that are overly acidic will also help stomach conditions. Any cooked or processed food puts strain on your digestive system. These foods simply do not have enough raw enzymes and nutrients to aid in digestion. It would be wise to eat at least half of all of your meals as raw or steamed veggies. This will give your body some support in breaking food down and help with reducing the potential for heartburn. I would also recommend taking digestive enzymes with all your meals.

Digestive enzymes taken with your meals will drastically reduce your heartburn symptoms and will also help with absorbing nutrients better. Most people are deficient in enzyme levels in their bodies, so it is wise to make this a daily practice with all main meals. Enzymes are very important for your overall health. Not all digestive enzymes are beneficial to use. You need to know what you are looking for because it is important to take an enzyme that works as intended. There are many brands of enzymes out in the markets. I would strongly recommend taking ones that contain only natural fruit and vegetable enzymes.

Holistic & Safe Weight Reduction

There have been so many diet programs and weight reduction devices over the years. Most weight reduction programs will not help you to lose weight permanently. It is quite evident that most weight reduction diets, strategies and supplements are not effective at helping overweight people to experience lasting results, would you agree?

I am going to educate you on the real solution to being slim and healthy. It does not involve crazy diets or spending hours a week doing cardio. These means of weight reduction are not effective and in fact can be quite dangerous to your health. When you know the proper information, this is when you experience results. In fact, the permanent solution to weight reduction is so simple that you will be amazed.

First of all, engaging in restrictive diets such as reducing calories and fat is actually counterproductive. The reality is that you may be causing your body to become fatter in the end. How are you doing this? Your body requires fat for numerous functions. It is an important compound for all overall health. The issue of today is the types of fats that people are ingesting, mainly hydrogenated fats.

These are the types of fats that are seriously harming people. Also, the consumption of excess empty carbohydrate foods such as pasta, white bread and sugar contribute to weight gain. These foods cause imbalances in blood sugar levels and body chemistry which in turn can cause weight gain.

Reducing calories and fats from your diet may actually program your cells to store more fat on your body. You have a mechanism in your body that is responsible for burning calories and fat. This divine mechanism is called the Basal Metabolic Rate. It determines how fast your body burns calories. You can alter your Basal Metabolic Rate quite easily. In essence, a high metabolic rate will burn calories and fat much faster. A slow metabolic rate will burn calories and fat much slower.

Lean muscular type people will tend to have high Basal Metabolic Rates. This means that their bodies burn calories much quickly and more efficiently than someone with a fuller frame body which has a slower BMR. The key to weight reduction is learning to increase your BMR naturally without stimulants and drugs. Most weight reduction programs stimulate your nervous system and are not healthy for permanent and safe weight reduction. Dieting and restricting calories and fats actually causes you to shift your BMR to burn much slower because it puts your body in survival mode since it thinks it is not being fed in proper quantities for health. This is a natural survival mechanism of a human body and thus millions of people are doing this to their body every day. Thus, you have millions of overweight people. Visit my website to view my Body Brilliance Holistic Slimming Makeover Multi-Media Kit.

Most People are Carrying Toxins

Your body will always seek to protect you from potential harm. Your organs are the most important components of your health. Thus, your body has a divine mechanism to ensure that your organs always get protected first. When you eat foods that contain numerous chemicals in them, your body has to deal with these toxins in some fashion. Excess toxin consumption will not allow your body to function optimally. Thus, these toxins get stored inside your body and cells.

As I have already said, your body will always protect your organs first. In the attempt to protect you from the toxic compounds that you ingest, your body will neutralize these toxins so that they cannot cause you harm. How does your body neutralize the toxins? It produces fat globules around them. As you continue to accumulate toxins, the body continues to form fat globules around them. The body will also draw these fat deposits away from the organs as to protect them completely.

These deposits usually get stored in the legs, waist area, hips and buttocks. Again, this is the body's attempt to protect you from the harm of the toxic chemicals that you are ingesting. The more processed foods you eat, the more toxic internally you become. This causes your body to create fat globules to neutralize the toxins. In actuality, this is a perfect mechanism. Your body is only performing its duty.

Most obese people are literally starving for nutrition. Their bodies are so toxic and nutrient deficient. If you look at the diets of many overweight people, you will find in most cases that they are ingesting high quantities of toxic foods. So, the real issue with weight gain is chemical in nature. There are times when weight gain can be attributed to mental and emotional dysfunction. There can be subconscious factors that would cause a person to gain weight and hold onto it.

At times a person may feel the need to be protected. Subconsciously, the mind will trigger bio-chemicals that are responsible for storing weight on the body. Your subconscious mind equates fat with protection. So, if a person experienced some kind of trauma that caused them to feel they were hurt, abused, or humiliated, then this may set up a subconscious defense for protection (fat).

The True Solution To Permanent & Safe Weight Reduction

The simple solution to losing excess body weight, and keeping it off permanently, is to stop eating foods that contain toxic ingredients and also sweetened drinks and all forms of processed sugars. You also require to get rid of the toxins out of your body. You then require eating a balanced and wholesome diet for your body type.

Get rid of the toxins and you get rid of most of the fat that is around those toxins. Engaging in an extensive detoxification program can dramatically improve your health and help you to reduce weight permanently and safely. It is critical to learn how to detoxify your body in the appropriate manner. This will ensure the most effective weight reduction benefits. Obviously, a balanced regimen of detoxification and mental and emotional cleansing will compound the benefits you receive.

Consumer Beware

There are hundreds of food products that contain MSG in them. In fact, I would bet that at least 50% of the food you see in most grocery stores will contain MSG in some form. Again, the name may be disguised as some other term, however, it is MSG. Here's a little hint: Many of the foods that are processed and are in pre-made packages may contain MSG…foods like chips, frozen meals, sauces, lunch meats and many others. Fast food restaurants use MSG in most of the foods they prepare. Do you seem to have a craving for certain fast food at times? Or how about the strong craving for your favorite chip or snack food? I will bet that it is the MSG that had caused you to become addicted to that food item. The expression of: "I bet you can't eat just one" comes to mind when talking about this subject. MSG can be as addicting as any drug.

Why do you think that the United States has the highest percentage of overweight people? It is because many of the packaged foods have MSG causing people to become addicted to them, meaning they will eat more per serving and buy them more frequently. Eliminate foods with MSG and other unhealthy compounds in them and watch what happens to your weight and your health! It is simple. What do you choose?

You will gain weight easily by ingesting the following compounds

Corn Syrup – any time you ingest anything with corn syrup, the physiological effect on your body is that your system will convert this right to fat because of the molecular structure to the sugars. You will gain more weight by drinking soda or any other sweetened drink than food. Beer also causes rapid weight gain since it gets converted to sugar in your body and then gets converted to fat. Beer also promotes the growth of parasites. You will also gain weight easily every time you ingest anything with processed sugar. Processed sugar is not meant to go in the body. It is actually quite toxic to your system. The molecular structure and composition to the sugar is not healthy and actually degenerates the body and can alter your hormone levels. It makes your body acidic and stimulates your nervous system. It gives you a false energy by stimulating your brain and nervous system. So, in actuality, consuming any processed forms of sugar depletes you of energy and nutrients because of the physiological effect on the body.

Again, sugar is toxic to your system and thus your body attempt s to neutralize the toxic effects. Sugar also promotes the growth of parasites and yeast (fungi). Many people of today have lots of parasites which in turn put out their own toxins into your system which in turn may cause more weight gain. As I have already revealed, your body produces fat globules around toxins to neutralize them from doing your organs harm. Parasites can also cause your brain chemistry to be altered and they may even cause you to crave specific sweet foods. Parasites feed off of processed sugars of any form. They contribute to making your system toxic and may cause you weight gain or at least make losing weight a challenge.

White flour products also contribute to weight gain. These foods contain no nutrients other than starches which in turn break down into sugars in your body when you ingest them. Did you get that? By eating white flour products, the physiological effect on your body is that your system will convert it to sugar which then gets converted to fat in your body. Many white flour products also contain sugar as an ingredient which makes that food product a double whammy because you have in actuality a product of high dose sugar once you ingest it. Both will get converted to fat in your body. These foods also promote parasite growth since the flour gets converted to sugar once in your body. Again, this is a cycle that is self-feeding as long as you keep ingesting high sugar, white flour, and low quality foods and drinks. You require getting off the cycle completely if you want any resolution whatsoever. Consuming drinks that are sweetened will cause you to put on weight easily as well.

If you can remove just 2 compounds from your diet, you will immediately feel the difference. Removing white flour products and any and all products that contain any form of processed sugars shall do wonders to your health and shall make losing weight much simpler.

Vaporizing The Fat Off Your Body – The True Solution You Have Been Waiting For

The time has come for you to take a stand and begin your path to wellness, to a healthier and slimmer you. Are you ready? Great! I am now going to lay out the foundation of what you must do to experience the resolution and the results you have been wanting. These are actually quite simplistic, however, because you have been programmed to believe otherwise, it may take a bit of time for you to embody and believe the following knowledge. Keep in mind that you have been following habits for some time now, so it shall require consistent conscious awareness and the intention to keep progressing. As you continue to be consistent with your intentions while also being conscious of the path you are following, this creates a powerful synergy that compounds and gets results. The results you experience are determined by you and how far do you want go and how healthy and radiant do you want to be? Getting the results you desire are absolutely attainable, however, the question is…are you willing to walk the path to getting there? That is something only you can say.

To begin your path to a healthier and slimmer you, I recommend to begin sitting with yourself and write down any and all feelings of unresolved life issues. It usually is one or more people that you have issues with. In some way they did or said something that impacted you. The feelings about those people require to be addressed because they may be the contributing factor to your being overweight. Many people tend to ingest sugary and salty foods in the attempt to numb over these inner feelings in a subconscious manner. So, write down what you think those feelings are, is it sad, is it angry, is it confused. Write them down. Next, begin to talk to these feelings as if they are a person. Ask them what they want and what can you do to help them to express themselves. Write down what comes. Sometimes simply honoring the feelings and just allowing them to express themselves resolves them and you begin to feeling better.

Give it a try and see. The main point here is that the unresolved inner feelings require being expressed and transformed because they are the root and if you want lasting results and fantastic health levels then this process is essential. Do this process for a few weeks on a daily basis and see what shifts may occur for you. You can always say that you love them (the feelings) and honor them. Give your feelings acknowledgment and learn to listen to what they are teaching you. Sometimes they will reveal some real powerful life wisdom that can help you in many areas of life. Become a student of your inner self because there is some powerful knowledge and wisdom in there. You will be surprised at what you learn when you are sincere and honest with doing this work.

The next step on your path to a healthier and slimmer you is to begin eliminating the foods and drinks that are contributing to your weight issues. This is a process that requires to be done properly because to eliminate only a few items is not going to get you results as you have already proven to yourself. In essence, you require a whole nutrition and lifestyle makeover. In order for you to get lasting results then you require to follow nutrition intake and a lifestyle that supports those results. So, the main foods and drinks to eliminate are: all white refined food products, all food products containing processed sugar in any form including corn syrup, cane juice, powdered sugar, and fructose.

White pasta and white rice are foods to eliminate as well as these get converted to sugar in your body. Also eliminate all sweetened drinks and alcohol such as beer, wine and liquor as these get converted to sugar in your body which then get converted to fat. Drink kombucha or coconut water kefir instead. Also eliminate all foods that contain any of the refined oils such as canola, corn, vegetable, margarine, soybean, Crisco, and any other hydrogenated oil as an ingredient. These oils make your body toxic and can also contribute to weight gain.

The next step is incorporating the foods that will supply you with nutrients and will help with vaporizing the fat off your body. The following food groups are essential in your life makeover: wholesome foods such as fresh vegetables and fruits, high quality oils as in coconut oil, grapeseed oil, Organic pure olive oil, sprouted nuts, almond butter, cashew butter, and tahini, sprouted whole grain breads, whole grain gluten-free flours, select portions of fatty meats as in free-range chicken legs and wings, free range rib eye steaks and ground beef, lamb, and Alaskan salmon. The fatty portions of meat are actually the healthiest to eat, they are easier to digest and contain healthy fats that you require for a healthy body. These fats will also help you to lose weight effectively in conjunction with the other daily habits you embody.

You require learning how to structure your nutrition intake properly as to get maximum results. You also require eating at proper times for your body type and lifestyle. My recommendation is to eat at least 3 holistically structured meals per day with at least one piece of fruit as a mid-day snack. This ensures supplying your body with adequate nutrients and protein to help with your weight goals. Each meal requires to be structured as to provide a balance of fats, proteins and carbohydrates.

For example, a holistically structured meal is the following: half of your plate (50%) ought to be a vegetable of some kind for every meal, the other half of your plate then gets a half (25%) of protein and the other half (25%) is a complex carbohydrate. This is a balanced meal and is the healthiest way of eating since vegetables contain minerals and fiber for regularity, the protein food supplies you with amino acids for rebuilding and the complex carbohydrates supply you energy. You require including a healthy fat in this meal so thus you can add grapeseed oil or coconut oil, butter or olive oil to your steamed veggies or brown rice. The oil fat will also supply your body with energy and shall help to give you lasting energy and strength throughout the day.

Super Health Foods For Optimum Health

The following food groups are the healthiest way of eating to ensure you receive adequate nutrient supply.   Sprouted whole grain foods, fresh pressed oils as in olive oil, grapeseed oil, coconut oil, avocado and avocado oil, almond oil, walnut oil, palm oil and butter, fresh nuts of all kinds, free range dairy and select meats. In fact, butter is one of the healthiest compounds you can ingest. It contains natural sources of Vitamin A and Vitamin E and other healthy fats that make this a super awesome selection. You can even use butter as a supplement by ingesting a few small slivers in the morning before breakfast. Your hair and skin will love it. Try it and see!

Fresh fruits as in local peaches, local cherries, pomegranate, persimmon, pears, kiwi, mango, papaya, star fruit, apples, blueberries, strawberries, raspberries. Goji berries are one of the most amazing fruits on the planet so be sure to purchase the best quality berries you can find. Eating goji berries on a consistent basis will do wonders to your health. Sea Buckthorn is also a life extending food and will do wonders for your skin and hair.

Sprouted whole grain breads and instant oatmeal are a great food to use for your nutrition. These contain complex carbohydrates, fiber and high protein and they are yummy. You may add soaked nuts and fresh fruit to make a healthy homemade cereal. Gluten-free oatmeal is also a healthy option, just be sure to add some protein and coconut oil and spices as in cinnamon, nutmeg and a dash of sea salt. I have a yummy recipe for oatmeal in my Fun Food Fantastic Recipe book called Heavenly Oatmeal. You can go to Amazon or my website to purchase it.

For natural sweeteners, you may use the following: a splash of yacon syrup, palm sugar, pure raw honey.

Free ranges eggs, raw cheese, goat yogurt, goat cheese, free range chicken (legs, wings, inners, thighs), free range beef (rib eye, 20% fatty ground beef, ribs), lamb, turkey legs and wings, Alaskan Salmon.

Organic nuts are an excellent source of healthy fats and proteins. However, you require soaking nuts before ingesting them as they contain enzyme inhibitors on their skins. You do this by placing nuts into a glass bowl and covering them with water for 6 to 8 hours. This will ensure that most of the funny stuff comes out, you then simply discard the water and now you may eat them for a healthy snack.

Baked goods may be prepared using gluten-free flours as in brown rice flour, sorghum flour, teff flour, quinoa flour, millet flour and oat flour, almond flour. Gluten is a compound that is in most hybridized grains as in whole wheat, rye, barley and is not healthy to the human body. It may cause a number of disorders so it is wise to either limit or eliminate this ingredient from your diet. Essentially, grains need to be soaked and sprouted before consuming them, however in modern times this does not really happen for a number of reasons.

So, most wheat products out there are not healthy for human consumption for numerous reasons. One, they contain gluten which is not conducive to health, two they are not sprouted, three wheat tends to get moldy and is actually the main cause for why some people do not do well with these grain foods. Mold is one of the most toxic compounds on the planet. It can really do a number to your health so it is wise to eliminate foods that are made with hybridized wheat ingredients. Use the gluten-free grains as these are much better on your body and easier to digest. You may require exploring with the gluten free ingredients a bit, however, you will feel the difference. Happy Baking!

The Future of Food Is Here – Super Nutrient Power Foods

There is one topic that many people seem to be unaware of and that is the foods grown in the soils of today are quite deficient of key nutrients. This is due to over-farming and the use of inappropriate agriculture methods that actually deplete the soil and the living bacteria eco-environment. The main point to be aware of is that most farms in this country have low level nutrient soils. This in turn means that the foods growing in those soils are going to have low nutrient quantities. For you this means that you are not nourishing your body for optimum health as you will require eating large quantities of food to ensure meeting your daily nutrition requirements. In essence, to receive your optimum daily nutrition requirements you will have to eat a large quantity of food every day. You may not be able to eat this much food and this can be quite expensive.

So, what is the solution? Actually, there are 2 super awesome ways of getting foods that are super high nutrient content. In fact, the future is to have foods that are super loaded with nutrients and where you require eating less to receive your daily nutrition requirements. The methods I am speaking to you about are growing foods hydroponically and aquaponically. In essence, this is the process whereby you grow vegetables in a liquid nutrient medium as opposed to using soil. These 2 processes are far superior to soil farming as they conserve resources, mainly water because they only use 10% at most of the water that soil farming does.

The good news is that these methods of growing food is the most efficient way of ensuring you receive the proper levels of nutrients. Also, the fact that these methods are quite simplistic to utilize and low cost to maintain compared to soil farming. Soil farming uses way too many resources to get a return whereas the hydroponically grown produce uses minimal resources and is super healthy for human consumption as the foods contain high levels of key nutrients. This translates into you be able to fully nourish your body for optimum health and longevity. Your body requires key nutrients every day, so to ingest foods that are fully loaded with these nutrients are going to make a huge difference in your health levels. To maintain high nutrient consumption daily is a secret key for living a healthy and long life. **Happy Hydroponics!**

You Must Learn To See Through The Veils of Illusion To Get To The Truth

EMF's & Their Impact On Your Wellbeing

The following information may or may not be new to your ears. I would bet that this will be the first time that you hear of it though. This is a key piece of knowledge to know if you are ever to restore your health. I am talking about electromagnetic frequencies in the environment. What's that you say? To explain it in simple terms, you can be affected energetically by electromagnetic frequencies and/or the energies of the people around you. This can cause you to experience symptoms of some kind and affects your health negatively.

What most people do not realize and what is not really being revealed in most instances, is that there are many electromagnetic frequencies in our environment that are harming your health. There are numerous devices and technological equipment that emit harmful frequencies. Devices such as cell phones, TV's, radio stations, satellites, microwave ovens, computers, cell phone towers, nuclear power plants, underground military bases and other frequency emitting structures can have a serious detrimental effect on your health. They emit frequencies that are not conducive for health.

Some of these frequencies can and do suppress the immune system. However, they can also disrupt other biological processes and cause a number of symptoms such as mood swings, headaches, nerve disorders, irritability, lack of concentration, anxiety and other health disorders. Some people are not affected too much by these energies in our environment. However, when you have a suppressed immune system, they can be quite harmful to you. In fact, it is critical to diminish or remove as many of these disturbing frequencies from your immediate environment if you want to have a full recovery.

These electromagnetic frequencies can put more stress on your immune system and can contribute to more fatigue and other symptoms as mentioned earlier. For example, you may be affected by cell phone frequencies, so when you use a cell phone you may feel more tired. Perhaps when you use your computer, you tend to feel more drained. When you are sensitive to an electromagnetic frequency you tend to have less energy when you are exposed to them.

It would be in your best interest to determine if you are being affected by EMF radiation. You can do this by simply observing how you feel when you are around certain devices. Notice how you feel when you are using your computer, cell phone, when you watch TV, when you use the microwave, etc. Make a note of it and you will find which ones affect you. I would highly recommend that you stop using a microwave oven. Microwave ovens radiate your food and change the molecular structure of the nutrients in food making them carcinogenic. When you are chronically sick, the last thing you want to do is eat food that has radiation in it and has molecularly changed nutrients. Talk about feeding a fire. Simply don't use it.

The good news is there are a number of devices that can transmute these harmful frequencies. You simply place these devices anywhere in your home and even wear them in your clothes for more protection. These devices are amazing and serve to protect you from these energies. You can feel a big difference in your health simply by transmuting some of these energies that are in your environment.

How you are affected by other people's energy

Have you ever walked into a public place like the store and all of sudden your mood changed for no reason at all? Well, that is because you were being affected by the energies of other people in that place. You see, humans emit energy just as all living animals do. Actually, everything in the universe emits energy. That is another topic and another book. If you would like to learn more about how everything in existence is not only comprised of energy but also emits a unique frequency individual to that object then you can research quantum physics. You will learn some amazing information about the universe and how we interact with it.

As my example above of walking into a store and suddenly feeling different emotionally, this occurs more than you think. Have you ever experienced an event where a person walked into the room and everyone there suddenly changed their behavior? Perhaps it was at work and your boss walked in the meeting room. Did you tense up or feel different? Did others in the room get affected too? The reason why this happens is because you are picking up that person's vibration or energy that they are emitting. This energy can affect you in many ways. On the other end of spectrum...there are people that when they walk into the room almost everyone in that room lights up and become positively changed. Again, this is because the energy or vibration that this person is emitting is good or vibrating in a manner that is healthy.

When you are energy sensitive like a lot of people are, you can easily become affected by other people's energy. Simply being near someone who emits disharmonic energy can impact your health significantly. Why do some people emit good energy and other disharmonic? Well, it really is not good or bad energy that they are emitting. It has to do with that person's emotions and what they are holding onto. Negative minded people and people who carry negative emotions like anger, hatred, jealousy, resentment, fear and worry will emit energy that is of a vibration that affects people and the environment in a negative manner. Likewise, people who are positive, happy, confident, joyful, peaceful, loving, tranquil and content will emit energy that is healing and enhances the energy of their environment.

I am sure that you know of people in both categories, don't you? Of course you do. Now you understand how and why these people can literally change the vibration of a whole room. What I want you to realize is that when you are not feeling well or chronically sick, this opens the doorway for you to be affected by these negative energies easier than most healthy people. You have to become conscious of who is in your immediate environment.

If you live with someone who is always moody, pessimistic, and carries anger or any other negative emotion then you may be affected negatively. Is it your spouse, a mother, your father, a boyfriend, a girlfriend or your neighbor? Who in your life emits these disharmonic energies? It would be in your best interest to become conscious of who in your life emits energies that are impacting your health. Keep in mind, they are not responsible for your health. You are the one that is allowing their vibration to affect you.

Here is the secret: When you are balanced mentally and emotionally, then other people's energies cannot affect you. Why? Your vibration will transmute their disharmonic energies. However, when you fall into fear, anger, bitterness, resentment, and sadness you then open yourself up to other's energies. The secret is that you will attract to you all the energies that are of like vibration to your emotions and thoughts. I hope you understand how serious this is! Do you? You see, we are really like magnets and we attract to us all energies of similar vibration. So, if you are in a good mood, then someone's negative emotions cannot be attracted to you. If you are in a state of anger or any other negative emotion then you will attract similar vibrations in your environment. This will only compound what you are feeling. (A great book on this subject is called Positive Energy by Dr. Judith Orloff.)

I bet knowing this will make you more conscious of your moods, right? If you take a look at people who are loving, caring and positive, they seem to love life and are usually always pretty healthy, right? Then look at people who are miserable and negative minded. Their lives usually are filled with chaos and struggle and limitation. This is because they are attracting these situations into their lives with their vibration. Their external lives have to match their internal feelings and thoughts. That is how the universe works…it is law just like gravity. I want you to realize how serious your environment can impact you. Look at your life and determine who and what is healthy for you and what is not. You are responsible for your entire life. You cannot blame the other person for your feelings and health. You are the one who set up the vibration to attract this into your life. If you don't like it then you are the one in charge. You have the power to change your life at any time.

It is of extreme importance that you find ways to transmute all the EMF radiation that is around your immediate environment. Healing requires that your energy fields are balanced and free from EMF radiation. These disturbing energies make healing much more difficult so it is in your best interest to empower yourself and do something about it. My intention is to make you conscious of energies that may be impacting your health. This is serious.

Again, if you want to learn more about taking control of your energy and immediate environment, please read the book I mentioned previously.

Chapter 5

The 8 Royal Diamonds of Optimum Health

When you incorporate the following 8 Royal Diamonds into your daily health regimen, you can be certain that you will be providing your mind, body & spirit all the essential factors for creating & maintaining optimum health for life. Your body and cells are programmed for perfect health. You just need to provide the essential components to your mind, body & spirit and then let nature do the rest.

Your cells are highly intelligent and know how to keep you healthy for life. Most of the food, water and air you breathe are polluted with toxins and impurities so it is of great importance to help your body out in every way you can. It is the same principle in which your car requires gas and oil for it to run properly, so too does your body require basic substances for it to function well. It is actually quite easy to create optimum health once you know the right information and apply it into your daily health regimen. Keep in mind that you are responsible for your health and wellbeing. Do not make the mistake that millions of people do when they shift this responsibility to their doctor or healthcare provider. As you can see from the facts of what happens when you place the responsibility of your health onto someone else's shoulders...you end up confused and ill.

You are a master; you simply need to remember that you are. When you stand empowered from within, you cannot be led astray or deceived by misinformation as is the case in our society. I live by a simple saying... The Proof Is In The Pudding! Let life reveal to you the truth as it is law. Life will always speak the truth to you.

Look at our society and see for yourself what the truth says about the health of most people. If you wish not to become a statistic someday then I urge you to empower yourself and become your own master. Your health is dependent upon you and you only.

I highly recommend you apply the following 8 simple Royal Diamonds into your daily health regimen. All it requires is for you to become more conscious of your full being. Realize that optimum health entails a balance of mind, body & spirit. Without this balance, you can never be optimally healthy. It is futile to concentrate strictly on your physical health. Yes, you may feel good for a while; however, you will eventually sabotage your physical health with your toxic thoughts and emotions.

The best way for you to receive the most benefit from the following health system is to simply add one Royal Diamond per week into your health regimen. After 60 days, you may experience a whole new level of health. Make the commitment today that you will follow this simple health system... Your Body Will Thank You!

Optimum Health Is A Choice, What Do You Choose?

Royal Diamond # 1- Oxygen

Oxygen is the most essential compound that our cells require to function and keep us alive. The thing I find most ironic is that very few people are talking about the importance of oxygen and our health. To prove this point, what do you think would happen if you stopped breathing for 2 minutes? You would be pretty uncomfortable, right? How about if you stopped breathing for 3 minutes? Well, you would probably be out of here. So then why do most health programs and modalities neglect to mention this important compound? If oxygen is the most needed compound for our cells, wouldn't it make sense to ensure that you are supplying your body with the proper oxygen levels before you concern yourself with any other aspect of health?

Here are some facts for you to consider:

- Oxygen is the most essential compound of your cells.

- Optimum health always starts with high levels of active oxygen in the cells.

- Oxygen is the body's internal cleanser and best immune booster.

- High levels of oxygen in the cells helps the whole body function at optimal levels.

- Microbes cannot exist in a highly oxygenated cellular environment.

- Most people are severely deficient of oxygen in their cells.

- Oxygen makes all other nutrients function better.

Attempting to create optimum health without getting your oxygen levels up in your cells is wasting time, money and energy. Every cellular process and organ function is dependent upon you having ample oxygen in your cells. Without enough oxygen in your cells, all attempts at creating optimum health will be inefficient.

Did you know that nature uses oxygen and ozone to purify and clean the environment? It's true! Oxygen is the miracle compound of nature and of your body. Oxygen in your body helps to keep you healthy and vibrant. It keeps your immune system functioning properly and also helps to keep invaders such as parasites, fungi and viruses out of your organs and cells. Due to the deterioration of our environment, the oxygen levels of the air we breathe are not at levels that ensure our optimum state of health. The percentage of oxygen in the atmosphere has decreased significantly over the past few decades as a result of the increase in pollution and the destruction of our ozone levels. What are you to do about this and how can you increase your oxygen levels if the air we breathe is low in oxygen?

There is one simple way to increase your cellular oxygen intake:

Do deep breathing throughout the day. This is the fastest and most economical way to increase your oxygen levels in your body. It is effective; you simply have to make it a habit to incorporate this into your daily health regimen. I suggest taking 10 deep breathes at least 3 times a day. Something you can use is to do deep breathing right after you finish eating your meals. This will work wonders and help your health out tremendously. Expect increased energy levels and more vitality. This is certainly one of the best and cost- free ways of improving increasing your oxygen intake and improving your health..

Royal Diamond # 2 - Purified & Energized Water

Water is the second most important compound that your cells require for optimum functioning. It is the body's internal cleanser & transport mechanism for every cellular process. It helps to transport oxygen throughout your body and carries all the minerals, vitamins, enzymes and essential fats to your cells. Essentially, water is how everything gets around in your body. It helps nutrients get into your cells and helps waste matter to get out. It is of key importance to maintain the proper hydration in your body. This ensures all the metabolic processes are allowed to function properly.

Most people in today's society are severely deficient in water. If you are like most people then you don't drink adequate amounts of water per day. This affects all of your cellular processes and leads to many symptoms such as fatigue, lack of concentration, lethargy, poor elimination, heartburn, acne, dried skin disorders and much more.

How do you expect your body to function without the proper hydration in your cells to move everything to where it is supposed to? How do you expect nutrients to get into your cells? How do you expect your waste matter and toxins to be expelled as they should without having the right amount of water to serve these functions? Don't you always ensure that you have the proper levels of gas in your car? It is quite easy to hydrate the body properly. Keep in mind that this is a habit that you must embody every day and not just a few times per week or when you remember. You will be amazed at how much better you will feel just by increasing your daily water intake.

Here is fact for you: The human body requires approximately 1 to 1.5 liters of water per day for normal physiological functioning. I suggest drinking at least 2 liters of high quality structured water per day. This may sound like a lot to drink, however, if you sip water all day long you will see that consuming this much water is quite easy. Simply ensure you always have a water bottle in hand no matter where you go. This is one of the easiest and healthiest practices that you can do for your health and well- being. Keep in mind that most water sources are polluted with toxins. It is crucial that you drink only structured water.

Your intention is to put clean water in and have toxins come out of your body. You are defeating the purpose of creating optimum health if you are putting more toxins into your cells by drinking polluted water. Also, for your body to absorb water properly, it must have the correct molecular charge. Without this magnetic charge then most of the water you drink will pass right through you. Most of the water that you buy in stores and comes out of your faucet is not charged at all.

Do a simple experiment right now. Go drink a full glass of regular water. After ten to fifteen minutes you will have to go to the bathroom. When you drink structured water or properly charged water, your cells will absorb more of it and you will find that you will not have to go to the bathroom right after drinking it like you do with regular non-charged water.

Nature has the perfect water source. If you have ever had a drink of pure, fresh mountain water then you know how good it tastes and how good you felt after drinking it. This is because the water was properly charged and had natural oxygen in it. Unfortunately, most water sources of today are highly polluted so therefore it is absolutely imperative that you drink only natural spring CHARGED WATER.

You require the right amount of hydration every day as to ensure proper functioning of your body as to get nutrients into your cells and wastes and toxins out via elimination. What you may not know though is that simply drinking more water isn't going to necessarily benefit your health, especially for longevity. In fact, most of the water sources today are not the right kind of water that your body requires for health and longevity.

Your body requires a special kind of water for optimum health. In fact, this Sacred kind of water is the way nature intended for us to be hydrated. You simply require looking at nature and the Truth becomes quite apparent. You as a human being need water that is from a natural spring source as in a river or stream or some kind of running body of water. Pay attention because this is profound and can make huge differences in your life. Water in nature is constantly flowing and spiraling (Universal Secret) as it travels down through rocks and mountains. What has been discovered for many years now is that water that flows in spirals as in rivers, streams, mountains and other such environments has a unique molecular structure that is ideal for human health and longevity. Another important Truth of water is that it requires being alive and charged with energy. In fact, this is the most important component to water as this energy then gets transferred to you if you drink it. So, nature knows best and is the only True water source that your body needs for optimal health and longevity.

Nature is the only source that can provide this optimum source for hydration as water that spirals via rivers and streams picks up energy from the earth (earth is magnetically charged).

Isn't it so beautiful that nature has the secret keys to optimum health? My main point is that nature has all the keys that we require for feeling and looking our best. How beautiful. If you begin to look at life with new eyes, you shall see a new reality open up to you. There is nothing mysterious about health and wellness. It is so simple that you miss it because you have been programmed to think otherwise. When you have eyes to see, the Truth is right there looking at you. The question is, where do you go to find this kind of water. As you are aware most water sources of today are polluted. Bottled water has become the normal source of hydration for most people.

There are many bottled waters on the market today. Well, suffice to say that most of these bottled waters are not in a structure that benefits your health in the long run. First, these waters are no longer charged with vital energy and many have been filtered to remove most of the minerals and other healthy components. Filtering removes pollutants however it also removes healthy components to water as in the Divine molecular structure. In total, bottled water is ok to consume for a short time period, however, for optimal levels of health, well-being and longevity, you require the living charged water that nature creates.

Many companies are using reverse osmosis and/or distillation to process water to make it cleaner. There are also home units that you can use to filter water and make it cleaner for consumption. Well, again, even though you filter the water and make it cleaner does not mean that the water is going to be healthy for your body over the long run. Actually, what is being discovered is that by consuming reverse osmosis and distilled water for a long time can impact your health in negative ways. The health benefits being proposed in favor of such water filtering are not True other than the fact that the water is cleaner.

When you process water (filter) in this way you actually strip the electron charge from the molecules and thus create a lifeless (no charge) water. You also change the molecular structure to the water and now create a water structure that cannot support your health over the long run. This lifeless water can't get into your cells as nature intended. This also means that minerals are not going to get into your cells as the molecular charge to water drives minerals and trace minerals in. Another important component to properly structured water is that it helps to remove toxins and waste products out of your body. You need to continuously have toxins and pollutants being removed out of your body, otherwise, they accumulate and get stored in your tissues and organs which leads to improper functioning of your body.

So, you need the right kind of water on a consistent basis to experience a Higher level of health and also longevity. If you do the research, the cultures that experience great health and longevity do so because their source of water is from nature and Earth charged. It is quite simple yet you miss this simplicity because you are programmed to think otherwise. Simplicity is where it is at my friend. Keep it simple. So, I know you want to know how to get this water then if your only options are to drink bottled water or use a filtering system at your house, both of which are not healthy to consume in the long run.

There are a few ways that you can recreate a properly structured water supply. As far as our modern way of living, these are the only True cost effective and simple ways of recreating the molecular structure and charge to water to benefit your health. You need to be careful as there are many companies out there proposing that their water machine or product does this or that and has these health benefits. Well, most of these interesting water products do not validate themselves. I have done the research and have a small list of products that I will recommend for better health and longevity. These validate themselves and are actually much more cost effective than some of these so called great water products. The first way to create a healthy charged water is to use specific earth mineral products that help to recreate the healthy molecular shape and to infuse the water with vital energy. I have discovered a few cost effective ways to do this. You may email me or visit my website to learn more about these products. They speak for themselves and are a much better option to what you are currently drinking. **Visit MyBodyBrilliance.com**

There are also a couple water devices that work by restructuring the water via information or energy. I will have the science of this device on my website as to go into detail of how the water gets restructured and why it actually works better than anything else. If you want to discover more about water and its True components then my recommendation is to get the book by Dr. Masaru Emoto, Water's Hidden Messages. This book shall knock you outside the galaxy for what he has shown with his experiments. Wait until you discover what water really is, mind blowing! My recommendation is to begin using one or a few of these products as to begin consuming properly hydrating water. Before you begin doing anything else for better health, the foundation is to drink the right kind of water because it shall allow everything else to work better. Happy Drinking!

Here is one simple and free way of adding frequencies to your water. Simple hold your glass of water or bottle with both of your hands and send love and blessings to it. Do this for a few minutes and then drink it. You can also ask the Infinite Creator to bless and restore the water back to its Divine Perfection. Explore with these ideas and have fun. If you must drink water while traveling the following spring water brands are good to consume on a temporary basis, so do your best in buying spring water from mountain sources only like Fiji, Volvic, Voss and Icelandic brands.

Royal Diamond # 3 - Detoxification

I want you to understand how important it is to detoxify your body on a routine basis. In fact, detoxification of your body and cells is crucial if you want to feel your best and stay this way for life. Most people go wrong when they think that they can just add some healthy supplements to their daily health regimen and eat more nutritious.

Detoxification Is The Mother of Optimum Health

Listen very closely to the following information if you truly desire to experience optimum health and want to see the best results with your daily health regimen. Without detoxing your body and cells in the proper manner and on a routine basis, you cannot get to an optimal state of health regardless of the quality of supplements you take and regardless of how healthy you eat.

Detoxification is an essential part of maintaining optimum health. It is the same principle as when you take your car for maintenance every so often by having the oil changed, air filter, the oil filter and keeping the chassis lubed adequately. So too do the cells of your body require this type of cleaning and maintenance. You see, you can be loaded with toxins and chemical compounds. Simply by being alive in today's world with all the pollution and processing of our food supply, these toxins get stored in your cells and tissues. You have to flush these toxins out of your system otherwise they impact your health negatively.

Your liver is one of the most important organs you have. It is responsible for absorbing and assimilating your nutrients and keeping your blood healthy and clean. It has many other functions to help keeping you healthy and vibrant. Here is something you may not want to know: Your liver is crying for help and has been for years. Why? Let me explain! Your liver is a filter organ and processes all of the nutrients that go into your body. After so many years of eating poorly and due to pollution and toxins found in processed foods, your liver becomes severely congested and impacted with deposits.

Imagine if you never took your car in to get the oil changed or any other maintenance for that matter. Have you ever seen your air filter in your car after only 6 months without changing it? How about what the oil looks like only after 4 months? It is black, thick and nasty. Now, imagine if since the moment you bought your car you never once changed the oil, the filter or did any other maintenance that your car requires for functioning well. Imagine how black and gooey your oil would be and how clogged your air filter and fuel filter would be. You understand this, correct?

Well, this kind of situation is exactly what is happening in your body when you never routinely engage in detoxification. Your liver can become congested with deposits and your cells can become toxic with impurities that your body cannot function properly. If you could look into your body on a microscopic level, you may see all the toxins, viruses, parasites and fungi making a home out of you. In fact, you would be disgusted if you could see all the toxicities that you probably carry in your body. These toxins, parasites and viruses need to come out if you ever want to know what it feels like to be optimally healthy. Keep in mind that you have the potential to feel great every day. When you are clean from the inside of all toxins and parasites, you will have more energy and a feeling of such lightness; you will think you are in paradise.

The reality is that you (unless you engage in routine detoxification) are so toxic and loaded with compounds that are not meant to be in your body. Your liver may be congested and your intestinal and colon membranes are impacted with food remnants and impurities. Your body will use up a lot of energy in the attempt to neutralize all these toxins. If you are always tired and feel drained of energy then you can be certain that your body is full of toxins. Once you are in this state, it is extremely difficult for your body to get back to optimal levels. Actually, there is no other way to get back to optimum health besides engaging in an extensive detoxification program.

It is absolutely pointless to ingest high quality supplements and eat healthy foods before engaging in an extensive detoxification program. When your liver is this congested, your body cannot absorb the nutrients from your foods and supplements in an efficient manner. Also, when you are carrying many pounds worth of impacted fecal matter in your intestines and colon, your immunity cannot function at optimal levels. A big part of your immune system lies in your intestines and colon in the form of friendly bacteria. These organisms are essential for maintaining health by helping you digest and absorb nutrients, scavenging parasites and fungi and helping with excreting toxins and impurities.

It is estimated that the average person is carrying approximately twenty pounds of impacted fecal matter in their body. YUCK! Then you have to factor in all the parasites and fungi that many people carry and you end up with one extremely toxic body. How can you expect to feel and look good if you have all this toxic stuff inside of you? You can't feel good until these toxicities come out. Taking nutritional supplements in this state is to waste money and energy. You have to be cleaned out before these nutritional supplements can serve you well. You must have clean filter organs such as your liver, gall bladder and colon to be able to absorb most of the nutrients from the food you eat.

Taking supplements when you are toxic is like trying to add clean water to a pool that has algae and looks black in color. No matter how much clean water you add to the pool, it will never look sparkling clean until you remove the algae and skim all the gook out of it. You too have to clean out all the gook in your cells, liver, colon, intestines and gall bladder if you want to feel absolutely the best you can. You cannot side step this process or short cut it. You're just not going to find a short cut to detoxification.

Detoxification must be the first step in any health program; otherwise, you cannot create optimum health and feel the best you can. If you took your car to the mechanic and he said that your valves are filled with gunk and your fuel filter need changing, wouldn't you have this done? Or do you think that you would just let it go?

Do understand where I am going with this? I am attempting to change your perspective about your body and your health. You have to understand that your body is so amazing and immaculate. I think you, like most people have just never been taught how to honor, love and respect your body for the divine creation it is. It is in fact one of the most amazing creations in the whole entire universe. You have such a privilege to have a body. I think our society has placed too much emphasis on material objects and neglected to really understand what our bodies are and what they do.

Every second of every day your body is going through millions of biochemical reactions and doing it perfectly without your conscious thought to power any of it. Do you see the perfection of your body? When you cut your finger or break a bone, all of the needed compounds to heal that wound are automatically and instantaneously sent to the point of injury. You never have to add anything or do anything special for these wounds to heal, do you? It all happens as if by magic. And most of the time you can never tell there was ever any type of injury to begin with.

Do you see the divineness of all this. Your body and cells are intelligent and know how to heal you and keep you healthy. Again, it is programmed into every cell. Whenever there is any deviation in the divine blueprint of perfect health that you carry, your cells know it and respond accordingly. The issue arises when your cells and body are so toxic that your organs and immune system cannot function at optimal levels. This is the point where poor health begins and becomes a ripe environment for illness.

Detoxification can virtually alleviate almost all health disorders alone. Keeping the body and cells clean on a continual basis can also prevent almost all disease and poor health. This is the secret to optimum health and it is the way for you to feel the best you can. You must participate in a routine detoxification program if you desire to feel optimally healthy for the rest of your life. This process can be fun if you know how to do it. Essentially there are 3 phases to a detoxification program.

These are:

1) Clean Out All Of The Filter Organs, Colon & Intestines

2) Get Rid of Parasites, Fungi and Viruses

3) Reboot The Immune System, Hydrate & Nourish The Cells

The Health Benefits of Proper Detoxification are:

- More Energy

- Healthier Skin

- Stronger Immunity

- Healthier Hair

- Clearer Mind

- A Sense of Overall Lightness

- Permanent & Safe Weight Reduction

- Slow The Aging Process Significantly

Royal Diamond # 4 - Nutrients

Nutrients are the building blocks of our bodies and are essential for optimum health. Your cells need these life essentials on a continuous basis. Without a constant supply of organic & ionic nutrients, your body cannot function at optimal levels. The same way your car requires gas and enough oil for it to run properly, so too does your body require fuel every day in the form of minerals, trace minerals, vitamins, enzymes, amino acids and essential fats. These are the basics of health and of life. Supply your cells with the foundational elements of life and you ensure that your vehicle (body) runs as good as it can.

It seems that at the present moment there is a crisis at hand. You see, most of the food supply lacks the vital nutrients that our cells require on a daily basis. The soils have become so eroded and over used that the core minerals and other essential nutrients are no longer present. This means that the food that grows in this soil is also deficient in nutrients.

Essentially, most of the food you eat lacks the basic elements of life that your cells require for them to function at optimal levels. Additionally, we have genetically modified foods that have been introduced into the food supply. These food items may look like normal food, however, their chemical makeup says otherwise. Your cells can only absorb nutrients and compounds in their natural form that come from nature. Your body cannot recognize genetically modified foods. Their chemical makeup is different than the ones from nature. So, for example, a genetically modified apple is not as recognizable to your cells as is an apple that is naturally and grown in a normal fashion. One other area of importance concerning our food supply is that a majority of it is deficient food. How can one expect to live on canned and prepackaged food? How can a living cell survive on chemicals and substances that are toxic?

Go through any grocery isle and more than 90% of those items cannot feed your body adequately! Do you think that this is serious? Of course it is and yet not many people seem to be concerned. If you truly desire to feel optimally healthy, then it is crucial for you to start nourishing your cells adequately. Correct me if I am wrong, but, when the gas tank in your car is close to empty, you go fill your tank up with the right kind of gas, right? So why wouldn't you have this same attitude for your body?

Wouldn't it be more important for you to make sure you are putting the right kind of nutrients and foods into your body before you have concern for anything else? Your body is your temple and only you can put things into it or on it. Shouldn't our society place a higher emphasis on our health and what we put into our bodies than concern ourselves with what octane gas we put in the car?

I think our society is in for a rude awakening. Most people do not see the epidemic that is at hand. This attitude of putting material objects ahead of their health is a one way road to poor health and a shortened life span. I suggest if you do not want to be a statistic someday then you best empower yourself and embody what you learn about creating optimum health. The following is basic knowledge of the key elements of life and health. Learn them and embody them on a daily basis.

Minerals

Minerals are inorganic compounds that your body requires for numerous functions such as bone formation, healthy skin, immune support, digestion, eliminating acids and wastes out of the body and normal heart function. The key minerals that are essential for optimum health are calcium, potassium, sulfur, magnesium, sodium and phosphorus. Your cells use these essential components to keep you healthy and help your body function the way it does. As I already talked about, most of the food supply is seriously deficient in these key elements of life, meaning that you are not receiving the proper levels to keep you healthy.

It is imperative for you to receive enough minerals and trace minerals on a daily basis. Trace minerals are minerals that are not needed in as high of quantities as the key essentials mentioned before. It is of critical importance to modify your diet and use the proper nutritional products to ensure your body receives its foundational nutrients for optimum health.

When using mineral supplements be sure that the product contains ionic and/or angstrom sized minerals. Most mineral supplements contain colloidal or synthetic nutrients. These minerals are not suitable for your cells as their size and chemical make-up are not in a fashion where they can be absorbed easily.

Colloidal minerals are too big to enter into your cells. It is like trying to force a basketball into a golf ball size hole. It just isn't going to go through. Ionic minerals and angstrom sized minerals are typically many thousands of times smaller than colloidal minerals and are easily absorbed by the cells. Their chemical make-up and magnetic charge make these types of minerals the best possible choice for your health.

Oh, by the way…plants and fruits contain ionic minerals and in the size that our cells require for absorption. Remember this of all things you read here...**NATURE KNOWS BEST!**

One more important piece of information for you to know is that the reason why most supplements and health products sold in the public domain are not really good for your health is that they are synthetically made, meaning their composition or chemical make-up is not in a natural form and the way they are processed leads them to be poor quality nutrients. Most supplements also contain binders and fillers that make up a large percentage of the pill or capsule leaving you with only a small dose of actual nutrient. Some companies add coal tars and other toxic compounds in their products; substances which do not belong in the body nor can your cells absorb.

There is a lot of marketing hype out in the public domain about many health supplements. I would caution you to stay clear of the hype and concentrate on only the supplements that are of high quality and essential for your cells. Most health products such as multi-vitamins and other combination supplements typically are not as good as ones that have the correct ratio of nutrients and in the right quantity.

As I have already stated...NATURE KNOWS BEST! Natural foods like fruits and vegetables contain nutrients that are in the proper ratios and concentrations and are easily absorbed by your cells. The easiest and best way to receive your nutrient requirements is to eat whole foods in the form of raw organic fruits and some raw and mostly steamed vegetables. Juicing allows you to ingest larger quantities of nutrients without the bulk and without having your body expend excessive amounts of energy to break down the nutrients, however, my recommendation is to juice only veggies and keep the fruits out, they are too concentrated in sugars when in liquid form. This can spike you insulin levels and disrupt your metabolism.

Organic vegetables tend to have higher concentrations of nutrients since organic farming utilizes healthier agricultural practices by rotating crops and adding essential nutrients to the soils via various farming methods. However, even organic produce is going to lack vital nutrients for long term health. Thus, you must supplement with the proper nutrients that are pure and natural. Please visit my website for supplements that are life giving and validate themselves. www.MyBodyBrilliance.com

Vitamins

Vitamins are organic chemical compounds the body uses for cellular growth, repair and normal metabolic functioning of your cells. Understand that vitamins require that you have enough minerals in your cells to function properly. Think of it as a lock and key system. Minerals work along with vitamins so they work together symbiotically to help all the biochemical reactions of the body to function as they do, such as converting food into energy.

Your body can produce some of the vitamins it requires to function well. It is important to ensure you are receiving enough trace minerals and minerals first since the body has an immaculate capability to produce vitamins. Minerals on the other hand cannot be produced by the body and so require a continuous supply from the food you eat or through supplementation.

Enzymes

Enzymes are some of the most important compounds in the body. These protein molecules serve as a catalyst for almost all of the biochemical processes that occur in your body. In fact, without these important compounds you couldn't remain healthy. They are responsible for initiating key processes like converting food to energy, cellular regeneration, digestion, detoxification, respiration and proper immune function. Think of enzymes as the spark plugs in your car. The spark plugs in your car serve to provide the catalyst for your engine to start. Without this key process (spark) your car's engine cannot start.

If you do not have the proper levels of enzymes in your cells, then your body cannot function at optimal levels. When cellular enzyme levels are low in the body, key biochemical processes are not allowed to occur as they should, resulting in poor organ function which in turn leads to poor health. Most people are deficient in enzymes in today's society. As stated earlier, the food supply is lacking in the vital nutrients that your body requires for optimum functioning.

Enzymes are also deficient in much of the food supply due to over farming and poor agricultural practices. Another main reason why enzymes are so deficient in fruits and vegetables are due to the fact that most of the foods you get at the store have been irradiated which destroys the vital nutrients and enzymes in them.

Keep in mind that there are different types of enzymes required for your body to function optimally. There are metabolic enzymes, digestive enzymes, immune enzymes, respiratory enzymes, and hormonal enzymes, each having their own specific purpose in the body. It is imperative that you have the proper levels of enzymes in your cells. Optimum health requires that your body has an abundance of enzymes. Your body can produce its own enzymes; however, it only has a limited supply. Once these reserves gets used up then you have to supplement with the proper enzymes.

There are only 2 ways to increase your enzyme levels in your cells:
1) Consume foods that contain key enzymes. Eating food like organic fruits and vegetables, seaweeds like dulse, nori and kombu, juicing wheatgrass and barley grass is a great way to get your enzymes.
2) Taking the right enzyme supplements. There are many enzyme products available, however, only a handful of these products contain the right kind of enzymes and in the quantities that can help your body to function better. I

highly recommend supplementing with a high quality digestive enzyme. Taking digestive enzymes after meals can dramatically improve your health and well -being. Visit my website for holistic enzyme supplements. www.MyBodyBrilliance.com

Antioxidants

Antioxidants are an important category of nutrients that serve a key role in keeping your body healthy. Their main function is to keep free radicals from attacking your cells. Free radicals are unstable molecules and seek to bond with other molecules. This is where the danger lies as far as your health is concerned. Free radical can at times bond with cells, which in turn cause those cells to become unstable molecularly and open the doorway for poor functioning. Free radicals are formed in the normal process of many of the biochemical reactions occurring in your body. Typically, most free radicals are harmless to your health and in normal instances your immune system keeps the numbers of free radicals in check.

The issue is when the free radicals in your body become excessive in number and your immune system can no longer keep up with scavenging these unstable molecules. Not all free radicals are harmful to you. In fact, there are certain free radicals that are essential for your immune system to destroy parasites, viruses and fungi. Harmful free radicals can come from numerous initiating factors such as radiation exposure from cell phones, environmental pollution, smoking, eating poorly and junk foods, pesticides from fruit and vegetables, meats that contain synthetic hormones, chemical toxins in your skin care products and even the water you drink.

The diet of most people leads to the formation of free radicals in the body. Cooking with fats that are unhealthy such as canola oil, vegetable oil and corn oil cause free radical formation. Eating margarine and other hydrogenated foods cause the formation of harmful free radicals. Anytime you eat a processed food item you are causing free radical formation in your cells.

Antioxidants To The Rescue

Antioxidants serve as a key player in scavenging these harmful free radicals. It is vital that you always have a high level of antioxidants in your cells. Vitamins A, C and E serve as antioxidants that go about your body looking to take out any free radical molecules. There are also other compounds in the body that serve to scavenge free radicals such as Glutathione, super oxide dismutase and selenium.

Due to the fact that the food supply is so deficient in vital nutrients, it is absolutely essential that you ensure you receive enough antioxidants every day. Your body does produce antioxidants, however, only when you are optimally healthy can the quantities of these antioxidants serve to keep free radical in check.

Again, there are 2 ways to ensure you get enough antioxidants in your daily diet:

1) Consuming foods such as fresh organic raw fruits and steamed veggies and juicing wheat grass.

2) Supplementing with the right nutritional products that contain the proper quality and quantity of antioxidants.

Essential Fats

Essential fats or commonly referred to as essential fatty acids (EFA's) are an important group of nutrients for your optimal state of health. Think of this special kind of fat as the motor oil in your car. Without the proper levels of oil in your car, your engine will malfunction and eventually seize up. Essential fats in your cells serve numerous functions such as keeping your immune system strong, helping toxins to be excreted properly, helps the body to resist infection and also helps your skin to remain soft and healthy. These essential fats are very important for your overall health. These types of fats are also a good source of energy and in fact better than regular carbohydrates.

You are probably severely deficient in essential fats. Many health disorders arise when you do not ingest these oils on a daily basis. You must have the proper levels of essential fats in your cells; otherwise you are looking for trouble. Your body cannot produce these essential fatty acids on its own. You must ingest these EFA's on a continuous basis if you truly want to feel the best you can.

Most types of fats are not healthy for you to consume such as canola oil, corn oil, vegetable oil, Crisco, margarine, and the other highly processed (hydrogenated) forms of fat available at the market. Keep in mind that many food items on the shelf of any grocery store will have either one or more of (hydrogenated) processed fats. It is these types of fats that are severely harming people and even killing them. These types of fats are so processed and chemically toxic that your cells become severely impaired leading to poor health. Did you know that margarine is one molecule away from being plastic, as in your Tupperware containers? Do you think that your body wants this in there? Stay away from these types of fat...they are shortening your life span and can make you extremely sick.

The healthy types of essential fats that your body requires come from sources like olive oil, fish oils, grapeseed oil, coconut oil, avocados, flax seed oil, and hemp seed oil. You want to ingest oils that contain Omegas 3, 6 and 9. In my opinion, I believe that fish oil and hemp seed oil are the best choice for an oil that has a balanced combination of Omegas 3, 6 and 9. Flax seed oil is also a great source for Omegas fats, the only issue is this oil can go rancid really fast if it is not refrigerated properly. Hemp seed oil tends to maintain its freshness much better than flax seed oil. If you do consume flax seed oil make sure to put it in the freezer. In fact, you can put both flax seed and hemp seed oils in the freezer to maintain their freshness longer. These oils do not freeze when you put them in the freezer. Ensure that you buy freshly made oils. They have a stamp on the bottle that tells you when it was made. When you go purchase these oils at your local health food store please look at the label and see when it was produced. If the date of production on the label is more than 4 weeks old then I would not recommend buying it.

Look for a production date that is within 4 weeks of manufacturing. This ensures you are getting a fresh product. The best way to ingest these oils is to add them to a protein food source. A good recipe for the best absorption of flax and hemp oils is to combine 1 tablespoon of oil with 1 cup of cottage cheese and 1 tablespoon of organic fruit preserves. You can also add some fresh raw fruit like pineapple, strawberries or raspberries and mix.

Another way to add essential oils to your diet is to combine 1 cup of organic strawberries berries, 1 ripe avocado, 2 scoops of organic protein powder and 1 tablespoon of hemp seed oil in a blender and mix. Add some purified water to the mix to make it more aqueous. This is such a healthy shake and is loaded with fiber, protein, essential fats - Omegas, vitamins and minerals. You can use this as a meal replacement or a post workout drink. This shake is very filling and tastes great. Children love this shake as well and is a simple way for them get more nutrients into their diet. Try it and see for yourself. Your whole family will love it.

Royal Diamond # 5 – Sunlight

Did you know that sunlight is essential for your health? In fact, without enough sunlight exposure you would die. Your body and cells require sunlight for maintaining health and helping numerous bodily systems to function the way they do. Sunlight is actually considered a nutrient to some in the health field. It is responsible for creating a number of key biochemical processes in your body such as the production of vitamin D and other important compounds that your cells require for optimum health... Sunlight can keep your immune system functioning well and can even help to eliminate numerous skin disorders such as psoriasis and eczema.

In fact, all of life on this planet requires sunlight to live. Without sunlight there would be no plants on this earth which means humans wouldn't exist because there would be no oxygen being produced. Do you understand how important the sun is to all living things? The sun makes everything function the way it does. It is the catalyst for everything in our solar system. The fact is, you require sunlight in adequate doses for optimum health.

Again, I resort to the philosophy of Life Will Always Reveal The Truth To You. Sunlight exposure is essential for your health.

So, where's the danger then? Let me clarify some important points about sunlight exposure. You see, the danger of sunlight exposure arises from the fact that many people want too much of a good thing. The key for safe and healthy sunlight exposure lies in the duration of time spent in the sun. You need not fear the sun. You simply require the right information to be able to receive sunlight exposure and have it be beneficial for your health. First of all, being out in the sun every day cannot hurt you if you follow a healthy practice. For you to benefit from sunlight exposure the most, it is best to receive only short durations of exposure per day. Where people go wrong is that they want to spend all day in the sun and get a dark tan all at once. This is not healthy and can only lead to harm.

Staying out in the sun for extended hours of time is actually counterproductive. You will actually drain your body of essential nutrients and fatigue your system. The key lies in the duration of time spent in the sun. Staying out in the direct sun for 30 to 45 minutes a day is best. This allows you to receive enough sunlight for your health needs without draining your body of energy and nutrients. You actually energize your body when you stay in the sun for shorter periods of time and helps in the production of key vitamins like vitamin D.

I recommend staying out in direct sunlight for only 30 to 45 minutes per day at most. Listen to your body. If you are light skinned then you may only be able to stay out for less than 30 minutes - perhaps 20 minutes. You are your own master and only you know your body. Listen to it and observe and you will know when to get out of the sun. The key point is not to get any burn while out in the sun.

DO NOT PUT COMMERCIAL SUNSCREEN ON YOUR SKIN.

There are several reasons why you should never put any commercial sunscreen on your skin. Mainly, when you put sun-block on your skin, you will actually block the sunlight from penetrating your skin. This is completely wrong! Your health and wellbeing depend upon sunlight being able to penetrate and absorb through your skin. If you have a sun block cream on you will stop this needed process from occurring, which means your body cannot produce vitamin D, a super important vitamin.

Also, when you put on a sun screen, you will be adding toxic chemicals to your system. Sunscreens contain synthetic and toxic chemicals in them. When you add these creams to your skin they eventually end up in your body. These compounds can also clog your pores and block toxins from being excreted from your body. Your skin is a main path in which toxins leave your body. You want your skin to breathe so to speak to be able to allow free exit of any and all toxins wanting to leave your body. If you have blocked pores, you disrupt this natural process which in turn can lead to poor health by causing these toxins to be stored inside your body. Here's a doozy for you: You may increase your chances of skin cancer by putting a sunscreen cream on.

Another important point is that your eyes require sunlight to penetrate through the retina. There is a special kind of biochemical process that occurs when sunlight penetrates the retina and hit's a part of the brain that is very essential for not only eye health but also your total wellbeing. Wearing shades or sunglasses stops this process from occurring and is not good for your eye health. You will be allowing more sunlight in than is required which can lead to eye damage.

Here are some facts of life that I like to look at to determine if all the claims that are being made about sunscreen and sunglasses and the danger of the sun are true. I take into consideration the many cultures that exist still today that live in remote places and are in the sun all the time. I look at the people in the Amazon region, Africa and South America where these cultures and people live in the hot sun all year round and yet they seem not to be harmed. I look at the indigenous cultures like the Hawaiians and American Indians, the Aborigines of Australia and other cultures that lived in the sun all year round. I find that none of these cultures had an issue with the sun being harmful to their health. If you look at the facts, people started being harmed by the sun when health organizations issued warnings about the danger of the sun. If you do your homework you will find that there was a sudden increase in health disorders after health officials started issuing warnings about sun damage and people started wearing sunscreen and sunglasses.

Again, I always let life reveal the truth to me. The way I see it, people are harmed when they go against nature and listen to deceptive information. The sun is your friend and is essential for your health. You just need to follow a healthy practice of staying out in the sun. Here are some recommendations for you to follow that will ensure a healthy time in the sun.

1)   Only stay out in the direct sun for 30 to 45 minutes maximum per day.

2)   Ensure you drink plenty of water before, during and after sunlight exposure.

3)   Only wear natural skin creams like aloe vera, cocoa butter and plant based creams.

4)   Listen to your body. Get out of the sun when you think you have had enough. Some people only require 15 to 20 minutes of direct sunlight exposure per day. Again, only you know. Listen and observe. If you are going to be out in the sun for extended periods of time then you might consider applying an all-natural sunscreen after 30 to 45 minutes to protect you from burn.

Royal Diamond # 6 – Fitness

Fitness is an important component of your health. For exercise to benefit you the most, it must be a routine part of your weekly health plan. Only exercising once in a while or when you are in the mood will not give you results or benefit your health. Fitness training specifically has numerous benefits to your health such as the production of key hormones that are responsible for renewing and rejuvenating your cells. Fitness training can also have an impact on your neurotransmitter levels which affect your moods.

Fitness training also increases your energy levels and boosts your immune system. Moving your body is absolutely essential for keeping your lymph and blood clean as well. Lymph is the aqueous portion of your blood that transports nutrients and toxins to where they are meant to go. Your lymph is an integral part of removing toxins from your body and keeping you healthy. You have to keep this solution moving consistently throughout your body if you want toxins to be excreted appropriately.

At this point I will like to bring up the point of regular cardiovascular exercise. I am sure that you have heard for years that cardio exercise is good for your health and your heart. Well, once again, this may sound true on the surface, however, if you truly understand the nature of your body and how it functions then this immediately sheds light on the fact that most forms of high intensity cardio exercises are actually very unhealthy for you. Let me explain...your heart is already pumping thousands of liters of blood per day. It is on duty 24 hours a day. The last thing you want to do is elevate your heart rate for extended periods of time. This actually puts your body in a stress response, so in accordance, the body will begin producing stress hormones and is catabolic (degenerating, depleting). Humans are not meant to do long periods of any type of high intensity exercises. Short periods of exercise are ok to do, however, running on a treadmill, doing aerobics and running for long durations of time is not conducive to health regardless of the claims being made in favor of cardiovascular training.

Doing three to four days of fitness training per week is best for your health and well-being. Fitness training is anabolic (muscle building) and life enhancing. Your body will produce many wonderful life enhancing hormones by routinely engaging in fitness training with weights or machines. This is actually the fountain of youth people are looking for. It is already in your body. So, get started with pumping the weights, **Your Body Will Thank You!**

Royal Diamond # 7 - Natural Skin Care

Here is a simple fact for you: Whatever you put on your skin will eventually end up in your body. Did you know that most of the skin care products that you put on your skin are loaded with toxins and chemicals? All the products you buy at the store or pharmacy contain ingredients that are not healthy for you. Some of these ingredients are so toxic and harmful to your health that you would be surprised at how much better you could feel just by not putting these chemicals on your skin.

Here is an irony that you may find amusing, I know I do. Some of the chemicals that go into skin care products actually do the exact opposite of what the product says it does. For example, many moisturizing creams contain compounds such as alcohols, synthetic fragrances and preservatives that actually dry out the skin. Why would you put something on your skin that dries it out? You do this every time you put these toxic ingredients on your skin.

Go grab any of your skin care products right now and look at the label of ingredients. I bet you can't even pronounce most of them, right? There will be a long list of synthetic and toxic chemicals in there. Makeup, moisturizers, acne creams, lipstick, shampoo, gels, conditioners and even toothpaste contain synthetic and toxic ingredients that are not meant to go on your skin or in your body for that matter.

Remember, anything you put on your skin will eventually get into your body. Little do you know what kinds of chemicals that you have in your body right now from years of slapping these toxic solutions on your skin. Compounds such as mercury derivatives, alcohols, dyes, lanolin, mineral oils, toxic fragrances, preservatives, binding agents, and emollients are toxic to your cells and can cause a number of health disorders ranging from mild to severe.

DO NOT USE ANTI-PERSPERANTS OR SYNTHETIC DEODORANTS!

Anti-persperants block the natural expelling of toxins through your arm pits. Your arm pits contain glands that are responsible for excreting toxins and impurities out of your body. If you block this divine process, you cause these toxins to be stored in your body. This is the worst thing you can do. Toxins are meant to come out of your body and when they get stored in your cells and accumulate they could potentially make you quite sick.

Most commercial perfumes & colognes contain butane gas as one of their ingredients. Do you know how potent butane is? Well, it can act as a neurotoxin to your body and can cause numerous symptoms like fatigue, headaches, and even a dazed out feeling. Stay away from such nasty products. They can really do a number to your health. I don't think that your body wants butane inside your cells, do you? All the products you use on your body should come from natural sources like plants, seaweeds, seeds, roots and herbs. Natural skin care products also work a lot better than conventional brands because the body absorbs them better and has a better effect for your skin.

Most skin disorders arise out of toxins being stored in your skin and can show up as acne, blemishes and other skin abnormalities. Your body does not want or need these toxic ingredients. You have to understand that your skin is a defense system. Its main job is to protect you from all external threats. What you put on your skin directly affects your health. Do you want natural and healthy ingredients going in or do you want carcinogenic and toxic compounds going in? You decide!

It is my recommendation that you start throwing out your skin care products one by one. Start off with getting rid of one of your skin care products and replacing it with a natural version. Within a few weeks you will have a whole new set of healthy skin care products and your body will thank you. You may be surprised to find that you feel a whole lot better simply by using natural skin care products. Try it and see for yourself.

Royal Diamond # 8 - Emotional, Mental & Spiritual Health

The emotional, mental and spiritual components of your health are critical for your total well-being. In fact, they are more important to your health then physical factors alone. Science is just beginning to understand how these components of your being affect every aspect of your life. To experience optimum health, you require balancing mind, body and spirit for they are connected at the fundamental level. It is very similar to when you throw a rock into a pond; the ripples will eventually emanate out to affect the whole body of water.

What affects one level of your being automatically affects the other levels of your being, it is that simple. It is of great importance to learn how to incorporate a regimen that helps with balancing your mind, body and spirit. Without this balance, you can never be whole and healthy. Do not make the same mistake I did when I concentrated only on my physical health for many years until I wrecked my health with my toxic thoughts and suppressed emotions.

You are a multi-dimensional being with a complex psyche. You must attend to all aspects of your being to live in balance and harmony in life. You need to give attention, energy and love to these components of your being even though you cannot see or touch them. The magical part of who you are resides deep within your being. It is these invisible parts of you that carry so much potential and so much beauty. You have never been given the owner's manual of how to care for these hidden aspects of yourself. It is time to go deep within yourself and discover the Divine being you are.

You are not who you think you are. Who you think you are is an illusion that you have accepted as your truth. As you will discover as you go deep within yourself, you'll find the amazing being that you truly are. It is just like uncovering a gold coin while digging in the soil. The gold coin never loses it brilliance. It was just covered over by dirt for a while. You simply have to dig a little deeper to discover the GOLD that you are. It is there waiting for you to discover it. Only you can travel this inner path. No one can give you the directions of how to get there. This is a solo adventure that holds many blessings. You see, just like looking for lost GOLD, the process can be exhausting and confusing and at times even scary depending on the environment. However, when you finally find that beautiful GOLD coin, you realize all the digging and effort to getting here were worth it.

The inner path is the only way to freedom. It is the only way to experience the bliss that you seek. Deep at the core of your being awaits your GOLD! It is a decision that only you can make and it is a journey only you can take. Choose to discover the GOLD within you and you will see many blessings come into your life. Don't delay for the sooner you begin your journey, the sooner you will discover that all the things you have ever wanted for your life and the person you wanted to become were there the whole time. You will come to realize that there was never any need to become anyone, because you have been that and more. You just didn't see it because you have been blinded by the illusion of life and what you have been conditioned with.

Emotional Health

The emotional complex of your being is so important to your overall health. Your emotions are directly tied to your physical health every second of every day. What you feel emotionally always comes to the surface to reveal what is truly hiding deep within you. You cannot hide your feelings despite your best efforts to do so. In fact, hiding or suppressing your emotions is like holding onto to a bomb ready to go off.

The fact is that every emotion you have impacts your health directly. Every time you have a pleasant thought or feeling your body responds accordingly by producing a specific set of bio-chemicals to match your emotional state. For example, think about a time or event that was the most joyful and happiest. Perhaps it was an award you won, a goal you scored to win the game, a trip you took around the world. Remember those feelings! How do you feel right now? You obviously feel great, right? Now, think about a time that was horrible and scary. Remember your feelings. How do you feel?

This little exercise validates how your emotions affect your physical health every second of your life. When you have joyful feelings and happy thoughts your body is producing chemicals that enhance your wellbeing and extend your life. When you have feelings of anger, bitterness and resentment, your body produces chemicals that weaken your immune system and cause a number of health disorders. This has been proven by science. Again, I live by the saying…The Proof Is In The Pudding. Notice how you feel when you are angry or upset. Notice your posture and your energy levels. Also, notice when you are in a great mood, how your energy levels are and what your posture is like. For each emotion you have, there is a unique complex of chemicals that your body produces. Now that you are conscious of this you can learn how to shift your emotional states a lot easier by expressing each emotion fully.

The first thing you can do is simply acknowledge the emotion that you are having. Let it be there for now. Then, attempt to determine why you have this emotion. Is it bitterness, anger, jealousy or frustration? Then, let it express itself. It is like when a wave in the ocean comes onto the shore, once it has gone to a certain point it goes back out. Your emotions come in waves like this. Do not attempt to stop an emotion. Emotions are part of who you are and need to be expressed, otherwise, they get suppressed. When emotions get suppressed they become like ticking bombs. They need to be expressed; otherwise, they will come out in some way and often times they manifest as illness.

Emotions are real things and need to be treated as such. Simply because you can't see your emotions doesn't mean that they are not real. Emotions are energy. In fact the word emotion can be split apart to reveal this truth….E MOTION or Energy In Motion. Emotions have the power to heal or the power to hurt you. You decide which of these is to be your reality. Emotions are very powerful and act as a fuel to either propel you forward in a positive state or cripple you like tornado.

You must learn how to express your emotions if you want to be optimally healthy. Emotions can only hurt you when you remain ignorant of what they truly are and how to express them completely. Look at a child. They are masters of letting their emotions be expressed fully. When they are angry, they let you know. When they are upset they allow themselves to cry and whine until their emotions has been fully expressed.

Have you ever noticed when a child is crying or whaling? They remain in this state for a few minutes and all of a sudden it is like someone turned their power source off. How is it that they were crying so loudly a few seconds ago and then all of a sudden they simply stopped? It is because they have fully expressed their emotion. Once it is out completely then there is no need to continue.

By becoming more conscious of your emotions, you actually take some of their power away. Most often times you make your emotions worse because you want them to simply go away. This attitude actually causes your emotions to have a bigger effect on you. Here is a little secret you can apply that can dramatically change your life forever. The next time you have an emotion whether it is anger, jealousy, bitterness or frustration; simply acknowledge it for the moment. Say out loud, "I am now being Angry", then close your eyes and take 3 deep breaths. Concentrate on this emotion for a few minutes and thank it for being there. As you concentrate on the emotion, ask it why you are feeling this way. See what it reveals to you. It may be a word, a person's face or an event that happened in the past. Observe what is presented to you. Then, as you continue to breathe deeply picture the emotion being transmuted into a positive feeling like joy and happiness. Put a smile on your face and say…"I now feel great".

Acknowledging your emotions and letting them be without judging them will do more good than you can imagine. It will also diminish their power over you. Realize that ultimately you are not your emotions. They are part of your being but can only have power over you if you let them. Emotions are there to teach you life lessons. They are there to get your attention and point you in the direction of where you require working on yourself. If you get angry easily then somewhere deep inside you have anger stored. You are holding onto something from your past. It could be anger at a person, which is normally the case, or it can be anger at a particular situation that happened to you.

You are an emotional being so it perfectly ok to experience different feelings all the time. The harm arises when you do not treat your emotions with respect and wish they simply go away. The key is to become more conscious of your emotions and learn what they are attempting to reveal to you. Emotions are the way you experience this game called life. At times it will feel like you are on a roller coaster with feelings from one extreme to another. At other times you may feel more calm and peaceful. Don't judge your emotions when you have them.

You are human and life will always send you life events that will strike up different emotions from joy to sadness to anger to peace. It's ok, everyone on this planet experiences the same feelings in one way or another. The only difference is the circumstances that draw out these feelings in each person. Emotions make this game of life interesting, without them you couldn't have different experiences and feelings. Would you really want this? Life is about up and downs, peaks and valleys. It's all good. We humans like to judge everything and that is where our problems arise...In our judgments. Be grateful for who you are and what you have in your life. Love all of it because it is all Divine and Perfect!

Mental Health

The mind is one of the most mysterious elements in the entire universe. After all, do we really know anything certain about the mind? Where is the mind by the way? Most people tend to think that the mind and brain is the same thing. They are not. The brain is a totally separate entity from the mind. The mind is very mysterious indeed. I believe the mind is the bridge between our spiritual selves and our physical body. The mind drives the brain to function the way it does and in turn the brain carries out the instructions from the mind to the whole body.

Mind, body and spirit research is validating that it is a very powerful thing indeed. Your mind creates thoughts and these thoughts then help to shape your reality. Thoughts are energy just like your emotions. You can't see thoughts, however, they do exist and they do affect every level of your life, including your health.

How You Create And Attract Things In Your Life

Science has discovered that the mental programs stored in your subconscious are responsible for creating your reality. You may have numerous limiting mental programs running in your mind. The programs you possess will determine how your life unfolds and what you experience. For example, a person with a mental program that says they are not smart enough will sabotage their life in instances where they are required to perform some duty or accomplish some project.

Their mental program tells them that they are not smart enough so they will unconsciously sabotage the work they do on their project time and time again. Mental programs are just like computer programs. Computer programs carry out the same function over and over again without deviating once. They are perfect every time. Your mental programs act the same way and can cause you to experience all sorts of challenging and limiting life experiences.

Research has shown that children receive most of their mental programming by age seven. These mental programs then rule this child's life for many years and even into adulthood until the person changes the programs. These mental programs are very powerful and can make life hard if one is not conscious of them. Your immediate environment is directly affecting you every second of every day.

When you were a child, you accepted your parents' beliefs and assumptions about life. You then take on their beliefs and think and act in a similar manner that your parents do. This is called Tribal Programming. This is why you should be very careful of the environment that children are put into. Children are very easily able to be programmed. Their mind at this young age is very suggestible and easily influenced. You can get children to believe almost anything through repetition.

You are a victim of mental programming every time you watch TV or read the paper. You accept most of the things you hear on TV, radio and the paper because you believe them to be true. Here is a reality check for you: You have been programmed since you were a child and started watching TV and listening to radio. This is how people develop beliefs about all issues of life. They hear something enough times so they believe it is true even though it may not.

Typically, most people are prisoners of their own mind. They think that there is nothing they can do to stop the unending flow of thoughts coming from their mind. They believe the thoughts they have just spring into being without any source. The thoughts you have come from you. They come from deep within your being in the unconscious part of your mind or as some call the subconscious. This is where all your deeply held beliefs about life and yourself lie. I refer to this "unconscious" part of your mind just like an attic where people store all objects that they no longer want to see or use.

This is very similar to what humans do with old hurts and traumas they experience as young children. They unconsciously store all their wounds and beliefs of life into this compartment of their minds. These wounds and limiting beliefs then cause all sorts of painful experiences as they go through life because these mental programs are responsible for attracting certain life events into their lives.

The events that transpire will be symbolic or a reflection of the mental programs stored in the unconscious. For example, someone who experienced a lack of love in their childhood from their parents may have developed a belief that they do not deserve love. The mental program of "I Do Not Deserve Be Loved" will then become locked into their unconscious mind. As such, this mental program will cause this person to sabotage all intimate relationships. Regardless of how hard they "try" to find the "right person", deep down they do not believe they deserve to be loved, and so, therefore they get to be right every single time, even though consciously they want to be loved. The unconscious overrides the conscious mind in every case.

Your unconscious mind is actually there to protect you. It has in fact protected you many times in the past; you were just unaware of this fact. The unconscious mind is like your guardian and will always follow whatever programming that you have there. So, as a child you literally programmed your unconscious mind about many areas of life. The problem is, many of these old programs no longer serve you and at times can actually cause you to experience hard times in your life. These old programs have to be changed; otherwise they will continue to rule your life.

One example I can give you to illustrate this point is to use a belief that most children have when they are very young. In fact, you may have had this same belief when you were a child. Almost every child believes in Santa Claus. It gives children joy to think this bearded old man is going to deliver them the toys of their wishes if they are good. Now, for many children this is a good belief to have. However, a problem arises at a certain age when this child is wise enough to realize that their belief about a bearded man is not true.

As is normal, most children simply let go of the belief in Santa Claus. What were to happen do you think if a child continues to believe in Santa Claus after the age of 12 or 13? Do you see the problem? For a kid to believe in Santa Claus after a certain age would cause this child to experience a lot of grief in the form of teasing and ridicule form other children. Holding onto the belief in Santa Claus would clearly cause this child unneeded turmoil. This is exactly how unconscious thoughts and beliefs sabotage your life. You have to understand that you can consciously believe something and yet in your unconscious there may reside a belief that is contrary to this. Again, the unconscious wins over the conscious every time. Mind science has proven that whatever lies in your unconscious mind is the program that your brain follows, which, in turn is responsible for the life events that are attracted to you.

The events that come into your life are actually there to teach lessons and reveal exactly what thoughts and beliefs you carry in the unconscious part of your mind. They show you where you have limiting beliefs about yourself and of life. These life events are meant to make you conscious of yourself and where you require releasing old stagnant beliefs. As you begin to change your beliefs, your outer life changes as well to reflect your new beliefs. In essence, life is a mirror to what is going on within you. Look at your life and see what it is revealing to you. Where are you having hard times? Is it in your relationships, your finances, your career, your health? Life is always revealing your truth to you.

The key is to learn how to be more conscious of your thoughts and the events that unfold in your life. You may have many old beliefs about yourself and of life that are limiting. You must learn how to balance your inner self if you want the quality of your life to improve. This in turn will do wonders for your physical, emotional and spiritual health.

What do you think the difference between a person who earns a million dollars a year and a person who only earns thirty five thousand dollars is? IT ALL COMES DOWN TO BELIEF! Look at all the athletes and famous people who had rough childhoods, from being poor to having experienced traumatic times in their lives. How is that they have become so successful despite their hard times? Again, it is because they believed in themselves! Do yourself a favor and become more conscious of your inner held beliefs. Then look to change the beliefs that are sabotaging your life. This requires that you be honest with yourself and go deep within to find the true answers. One key to discovering your inner beliefs is to look at your life. How your life unfolds and the people who are in it is a direct reflection of the beliefs you carry. Look and you will see the truth.   **All The Answers You Seek Are Within You!**

Spiritual Health

The spiritual component of your being is very mysterious, wouldn't you say? People attempt to describe this aspect of our being with human words. How can you learn about something that is so out of this realm? How can you put into words exactly what spirit is? You can't! Spirit can only be experienced and felt.

All attempts to describe or define spirit will limit the profoundness of what exactly it is. Spirit is that mystical component of your being that requires you to delve into an unknown dimension. Spirit has always been and will always be mysterious and mystical.

Spirit is a magical essence that requires for you to discover it a little bit at a time. Without your spirit, you could not experience this game called life. All the answers to your life's lessons lie here in this mysterious realm of the unknown. Your mission in life is to learn how to access a direct communication with your spirit. Once you do, your life is never the same again. Your spirit is always waiting patiently for you to discover what you really are. All these years you thought you were a name, a body, a mother, a sister, a father, a son, a brother, an uncle and a list of other names that you use to define yourself. You are not these names and labels. You are something that cannot be put into words. You are something that is so immaculate and grand that any attempt to describe it will diminish what you really are.

You have grown up in a society that has never taught you how to honor and respect this component of your being. Man has created many rituals and processes in an attempt to acknowledge our spirit. These rituals do not truly connect us with our spirit. They give the illusion that they do, however, they leave us feeling empty and void inside. To truly connect with your spirit means to travel the inner journey into yourself. This is something that no one can teach you. It can only be learned and discovered on your own. This is a solo journey with no map to follow. The only thing that is certain is the mystery of spirit.

Your main mission in life is to merge with your spirit and become a whole being. Most people are disconnected from their spirit and so experience many trials and tribulations because they equate themselves to be the masks of life that they have created. Some people wear the mask of drama and some people wear the mask of the victim. Almost everyone has one or many masks they play. Which do you wear? Is it playing the victim? Is it creating drama? How about playing the dictator? Some people cannot exist without drama and chaos in their life. They have been so accustomed to experiencing hardships and tribulations in their life that they subconsciously desire more and more of it. These people cannot sit in a room for even a few minutes in peace and quiet.

If you truly desire to be optimally healthy and whole, you must connect with your spirit. This is the place of magic and is where all the peace, joy, abundance and happiness you desire for your life. This is the secret to life. All the things you seek and desire in your life can only be found in this mystical realm of what you really are. Society has taught you to seek outside yourself for answers to life's dilemmas. This is the wrong way. The second you go outside yourself to find an answer to your life issue is the second that you are going farther and farther from your solution.

Within is the only way to freedom my friend. No one out there can resolve any of your life issues. Yes, others can guide you, consult you and even inspire you, however, only you hold the magic answer to resolve whatever life issue you are dealing with. You are a master, for if you weren't you would not be on this planet. You possess an immense amount of wisdom deep within your being. Your inner spirit holds the map to create your ideal life. Your spirit waits patiently for your reunion. It is time to for you to become conscious of this divine part of your being. The time has come to shed all the masks that you have worn throughout your life. These masks no longer serve you and will only keep you bound to a life of limitation and illusion.

It is time to awaken to a magical life, one that is filled with joy, happiness, laughter, abundance and connection with others of like mind. This paradise exists in your heart already; all you need to do is bring it into your physical reality now. Your life is a direct mirror of what is resonating inside you.

Whatever you hold inside your being in the form of thoughts and emotions are the factors that govern what transpires in your life. The same way a garden sprouts forth whatever seeds you plant in it, so too does your life sprout forth what you have planted in the form of thoughts and emotions.

To experience the magical life you truly desire, you must plant new seeds, seeds of joy, happiness, connection, peace, calm and abundance. As you nurture and cultivate these new seeds you will begin to see a new garden unfold. All the solutions to life's dilemmas are there deep within you. All the desires of your heart can be had when you access the power of your spirit. There is no need to seek outside yourself any longer. You have everything you'll ever need in this life with you right now. All you have to do is take the inner journey and the magic will unfold before your eyes. I wish you many blessings on your inner journey.

All The Answers You Seek In Life Are Within You…The Question Is: Are You Brave Enough To Go Within To Go Discover Them?

Chapter 6

When Your Emotions Become Like Ticking Bombs

So, where does disease come from? How does it get manifested in your body in the first place? Do environment and diet really play key roles in causing disease?

Well, the information that follows will shock you to say the least. For years now health officials have told the public about how diet and environment specifically contribute to most illnesses.

Doctors have been preaching to their patients how important it is to eat balanced diet and to exercise on a regular basis. It is also advised to limit your fat intake because it is unhealthy. Many people believe that by taking vitamin and mineral supplements they will ensure themselves that any deficiency they have will be taken care of.

Well, although dis-ease is a physical manifestation, the root causes of most illnesses are not physical. The true root cause most dis-ease lies deep within every person that is ill. In essence, we create every illness that we experience, be it on a subconscious level or an unconscious level. So, how is that possible? How can we possibly cause ourselves these kinds of circumstances? Well, there are distinct emotional and mental patterns associated with most illnesses. The way you choose to use your mind and the way you respond to your outer world have more to do with disease than your diet and your environment.

We have heard in recent years how stress can kill you. Well, it is really not the stress in and of itself that will kill you, it is the way you choose to process the stress that could hurt you or make you very sick. The body in essence is a mirror of our inner thoughts, emotions and beliefs. Every single cell in your body has its own intelligence and is able to listen to what you are thinking and feel what you are expressing emotionally. In reality, your cells and your body respond to every thought you think, every emotion you have and every word you speak. Repetitive modes of thinking and suppressing negative emotions such as anger, resentment, bitterness, and hatred can eventually manifest as dis-ease in the body. Literally, your suppressed emotions become like ticking bombs waiting for the perfect conditions to detonate and manifest as dis-ease.

I hope by now that you can begin to see a deep correlation between your emotional and mental state and the state of your health. Whenever you have poor health or any disease, you need to look at yourself and see what you have been thinking or what emotions you have been suppressing. Many times though, the triggering emotional and mental factors for a specific disease occurred many months to even years before the manifestation of the illness. It is critical to discover the true root factors that triggered the manifestation of the illness. Even conditions such as the so-called common cold and the flu may have distinct emotional and mental factors contributing to them.

Any time you are sick in general, you need to listen to your body and hear what it is telling you. Instead of always looking for a magic blue pill or a magic supplement, it is best to be more conscious of your body. If you are chronically sick, then you need to assume full responsibility for your own health. No doctor or drug can cure you of any illness. You have the cure within you right now to eliminate any disease. Infinite Spirit equipped you with everything that you will ever need in this world.

How dis-ease really gets manifested in the body:

Symptoms of illness result from only the following 3 factors:

1) Toxic Thoughts

2) Toxic Emotions

3) Toxic Chemicals From Food

Your toxic (negative) thoughts cause you to have negative emotions. These negative emotions cause the cells of your body to create toxic chemicals. In turn, these toxic chemicals cause your body to create toxic cells that lead to DIS-EASE. Science is now proving that when you are in a state of distress and disharmony, your cells produce toxic chemicals that tend to deteriorate and degenerate the body.

TOXIC THOUGHTS > NEGATIVE EMOTIONS > CELLS CREATE >TOXIC CHEMICALS> TOXIC CELLS = DISEASE

Anytime you are in a state of stress and disharmony you then become susceptible to poor health. Also, when you are stressed out or carry any of the negative emotions such as anger, resentment, hatred, impatience, etc., you tense up. Tensing up in this manner causes many of your biological processes to be impaired. Nutrient transport, cell respiration, detoxification, elimination, digestion, assimilation, hormone production and brain function become severely disrupted leading to a gradual degeneration in your whole system.

Emotional stress has the biggest impact on your immune system above any other factor. If you are in a state of balance and harmony mentally, emotionally, and physically, then illness simply cannot set in the body. You have not been taught how to deal with stress and live in a balanced fashion. The society of today promotes drama, stress and struggle. The secret of how disease really manifests in the body is the suppressing and storing of emotions is the true root cause of most illnesses.

Diet and environment do help to contribute to disease; however, they are usually not the underlying root cause for it. Look at anyone who is calm and approaches life in a balanced fashion. These people rarely get sick and will almost never get chronically sick. Chronically sick people are ones that are typically very emotional and/or have had serious traumatic experiences in their past. They are also people who tend to hold onto emotions correlating to these past events. In fact, it is type A personality people that are more prone to becoming chronically ill than type B personality people. Which one are you?

What Is True Healing?

So, how does one begin to heal the emotional and mental traumas from one's past? The secret to healing yourself on all levels of your being is to learn how to let go and forgive. Learning how to forgive yourself and all the people who you perceived as hurting you is the best remedy for any life issue. Whether it is a chronic disease or an unhealthy relationship with a family member or past lover, forgiveness is the path to true healing. Notice that I said perceived as someone who hurt you. The fact is, no one can ever hurt you in life. You can only allow yourself to be hurt. The mental and emotional grief that you have experienced in life was really due to the perceptions that you had about each life event. The key is to learn how to change your perception of life.

I have found through personal experience that forgiveness is absolutely the most powerful healing force in the entire universe. I know that as I began to forgive the people that I thought wronged me, my health and my life started to improve dramatically. The question I ask of any person that says they are chronically sick or has any type of health ailment is...Who is the problem?

Forgiveness can actually heal you of disease. I will say that forgiveness is the magic cure that many people in life are looking for. You may be someone who is carrying hatred, resentment, anger and bitterness toward people you think hurt you. These emotions set in the body and get stored over the years until they manifest as disease and other imbalances. Your emotions also get stored in your energy fields and form blockages. There are now scientific instruments that can read your energy fields (aura) and are able to tell where you have energy blockages. Based on where you have energy blocks, you will be more susceptible to acquire certain diseases. In essence, if you can read people's energy fields (aura), you could tell where they are blocked energetically and be able to predict what specific diseases they are more inclined to experience.

Releasing old emotions can cause shifts in your energy fields and thus free up the energy blockages that you may have. That is why letting go of old STUFF can do wonders for your health. I have personally heard of people having miraculous cures of their illness once they decided to forgive someone. In fact, there are health promoting biochemical changes that happen in a person's body when they are in a state of forgiveness.

So, how do you forgive you might be asking yourself? Forgiveness is not some hard and complex process like you may believe. It does not take extended energy and time and requires no knowledge of how to do it. Here is the secret answer to forgiveness. Forgiveness starts with a thought, the thought of really wanting to forgive the person in question, letting the past event go and releasing the need to be right. The rest Infinite Spirit will take care of as long as you are sincere in wanting to forgive the person.

That is it! Pretty simple huh? It does work! Do it. The sooner you do, the sooner you will feel like a mountain has been lifted off of your shoulders. Not only do you free yourself but you also free the other person. Even if the other person never finds out that you have forgiven them, they will experience a release of some kind on some level. One bit of advice I can give is that to be able to forgive someone else, you have to forgive yourself first. The same principle applies here where you simply let go of the past, have the thought of forgiving yourself and release any anger or pain from the past event. In fact, I have discovered that the person we need to forgive the most is ourselves. Subconsciously, many people hold the most emotions against themselves and in turn this affects their health and their relationships. If you can really absorb the information that follows, you will be well on your way to healing yourself from whatever illness you have or poor state of health.

The Formula For Complete Healing:

1) Assume full responsibility for your illness. No one out there can ever heal you. It is your duty to heal all levels of your being to be completely well. By educating and empowering yourself with sound holistic health knowledge, you will be well on your way to healing.

2) Commitment; doing whatever it takes to heal yourself. Be committed to do whatever you have to do to heal regardless of how much money and energy you have to expend.

3) Forgiveness - as explained earlier will be the best remedy for your recovery.

4) Implementing a diet and environment that will support your physical health.

5) Learning how to adjust your thoughts and emotions to support long term health.

Holistic health therapies and true organic supplements can help you to heal on a physical level but only when you assume full responsibility for your health and become conscious of your full being. You are a multidimensional being with a complex psyche. You need to learn how to balance your multidimensionality. The only way you can truly heal from any disease is through healing every level of your being. You need to look at your mind-body-spirit complex and work to heal those areas that are out of balance. Without such balance, you can never truly heal!

Write It, Read It & Burn It

Here is a simple exercise you can do to help with releasing stored up emotions within your cells and your energy fields. Take out a notepad and pen. Think about someone that you have had any emotional turmoil with. Many times our family members are the ones that push our buttons the easiest. Perhaps you have some unresolved feelings associated with some of your family members. Pick one person that you feel you have some feelings stored about. Start writing a letter to this person. Write down everything you truly feel about them.   Keep writing until you feel you have expressed all of the feelings associated with that person.

Now, if you have a very close friend that you can share anything with then go ahead and read the letter you wrote to them. Tell them exactly what you are doing. They need not have any input. They are simply serving to listen to what you wrote, nothing more. If you do not have anyone you feel you can share your letter with then ask your higher power to listen to you and read it out loud.

When you are done reading your letter, go to a safe and secure place like a basement or garage. Get an empty bucket or some other type of metal container and put your letter in it. Now light your letter on fire with a match.

As your letter is burning, picture all the old, stored emotions that were in your body and energy fields simply being transmuted into positive energy. You are now free of these stored emotions. You should feel lighter. You may have to write more than one letter to one single person depending upon how much you have held onto over the years. The longer you have held onto emotions, the longer it may take to release the emotions. That is fine, simply be conscious of how you feel after burning each letter. Listen to your intuition and let it be your guide. Keep writing letters for each person that you have stored emotions for. Take one person at a time. Do not be in a rush to go through this process. Take your time and allow a few days in between new letters. Use this exercise and see how you feel. Let me know how it goes.

Happy Releasing!

AT THE SOURCE OF EVERY Dis Ease, LIES ITS CURE!!!

Chapter 7

The Greatest Longevity Secrets Ever To Be Revealed

You most likely believe that aging is a normal process and that all humans are subject to growing old as the years go on. Almost everyone has accepted this as a normal part of living life. As is apparent in watching family members and loved ones age, the human body goes through certain changes. These changes cause the body to look and feel different. Well, to say that I am about give you a whole new perspective about aging is an understatement. What I am about to reveal is going to totally revolutionize all concepts that you have about aging and growing old. Aging as you have come to understand it appears to be factual, that as you get older in age you look older. This appears to be true on the surface; however, there lies a secret that not many people know about. This secret will revolutionize what humans believe and think about aging.

What is this secret? Simple really, that your cells are programmed for longevity and can survive an indefinite period of time under the right circumstances. Let me clarify for you. Your DNA contains a blueprint for not only perfect health but also a program for your cells to survive for many years beyond what is deemed as the normal life expectancy of most people. Your DNA possesses the Divine blueprint of your whole body. It determines what hair color you have, how tall you are, the color of your eyes and even the shape of your body parts. Your DNA contains codes that serve as instructions for your brain to carry out. So for example, if you have a code in your DNA that is coded for black hair, then your brain will interpret this code and create black hair. The same process applies to all aspects of your body and health.

Now, where it really gets interesting is that you also have markers in your DNA. What are these markers? These markers (codons) act just like a light switch in your home. You can turn the light switch on or off. When you turn the switch to "ON" you get light. When you turn the light switch to "OFF" the light goes out. The markers in your DNA work in a similar manner. When these markers are "ON" they serve as a command to your brain to carry out specific functions. When they are "OFF" your brain disregards the marker and doesn't carry out any function.

In my previous example, your hair is a certain color because somewhere in your DNA there is a marker turned "ON" that is coded for this color. This is in fact how your whole body is formed…by the codes (markers) in your DNA. Now the interesting thing is that you can alter the DNA markers by turning them "OFF" or "ON. "

This in turn will give you a different result. Now, in the aspect of aging, there are codes in the DNA of each cell that are "ON" for you to age the way you do. Thus, your brain carries out the instruction to age your body. Now wait just a minute, because this is not a fixed factor. As I said, these markers can be turned off or on and in doing so you end up with a different result. What if there was a way to turn the "AGING MARKERS" in your DNA "OFF?" What do you think would happen? I believe the human body could then survive many more years than the average life expectancy. The Hunza people in the Middle East on average live 100 - 125 years of age, some have even lived to 145. They are able to live this long because they live balanced lives in the form of eating pure food, drinking pure mountain water and live stress-free lives. They have also come to expect to live this long due to their cultural programming.

Imagine what would happen if these people were able to turn their aging markers "OFF?" Yes, they would probably live to the age 200 or more. Do you see the possibilities of this unique perspective? If you are to study information on DNA, you will come to understand that DNA is not fixed as most people believe. The codons in your DNA can be altered. The question is how do you do this? This is the million dollar question. In fact, there are many scientists and research companies on a serious quest to discover exactly how to change the markers in the DNA for they see the huge potential. Imagine the possibilities of what you could do if you were able to alter your DNA coding. Science has already stated that it can be done. Expect numerous advancements in health in the coming years. I know this may sound a little too scientific but it is coming.

The 4 biggest factors that determine the rate of your aging are:

1) Stress: This has the greatest impact on both your health and aging. Tension causes impairment of biological processes and the creation of toxins in the cells which in turn causes them to age faster.

2) Unresolved Emotions: Suppressed emotions get stored in your cells and energy fields putting undue stress on all levels of your being. These emotions disrupt the normal physiological components of your health and affect mind, body and spirit. This added pressure to your being can cause the cells to age faster.

3) Internal Cellular Toxicities: The more toxicity you have within your cells the faster you age. This comes from eating too much cooked foods and foods that are overly processed which contain numerous preservatives and chemicals in them.

4) Belief In Aging: Beliefs are very powerful. Beliefs can cause you to experience a life of misery or one of bliss. You decide which beliefs to carry and it is these beliefs that shape your world. If you believe in aging then that is what you will experience.

Could aging be a mental program in your subconscious mind? Here is my personal belief; that it is the belief in aging more than anything else that causes you to age and grow old. Let me explain! Science has proven that mind, body and spirit all are integrally linked. They all function symbiotically helping you to experience this game called life. Whatever affects one of these components of your being automatically affects the others. It is just as a rock thrown into a pond, the ripple eventually emanates out to affect the whole body of water. The subconscious mind is directly responsible for the instructions that your brain uses to carry out all biochemical processes required for your body to function the way it does. The brain is like a super computer that carries out any function that it is inputted with. The question is where do the subconscious programs come from?

These subconscious mental programs come from you in the form of beliefs and perceptions that you have formed over the years. These programs can and do alter the genetics of your body. These programs then cause your brain to carry out the instructions perfectly. This is exactly how everything in your life is attracted to you and how you create your reality.

Beliefs + Perceptions >>> Form as Mental Programs In Your Subconscious Mind >>> Brain Carries Out These Instructions >>> You Attract & Create Your Reality According To What The Mental Programs Say

So, in the instance of aging, if you believe that aging is a normal process of life then this will get stored in your subconscious mind as a mental program which in turn will cause your DNA markers to be "ON" for aging. Your brain then carries out these instructions. You now get to be right…your body ages. Do you see how this works? In essence, the belief in aging gets passed on to the next generation which then keeps getting passed on…until there is a shift in consciousness. Mark my word, in 10 to 15 years time there will be a huge shift in the way people think about aging.

Psychoneuroimmunology (the study of how mind, body and spirit affects your health and life) is proving that almost all disease is caused by your state of consciousness.

So, yes you can and do alter the biochemistry of your body with your thoughts and emotions. In fact, you are doing this every day of your life. This is why some people age slower than others. Their mind frame and general attitude towards life determines how healthy they are.

We live in a world where everyone has their own unique reality based upon the mental programs that they have formed over the years. This is why it is so hard at times for some people to change their life. Will power and effort is not going to get results. You must change the programs running in your subconscious mind if you want lasting change and improvement in any area of your life. This is mind blowing stuff wouldn't you say? Quantum physics has proven that everything in life is just a state of consciousness and it is beliefs that create your reality. So, if everyone believes in aging then guess what, that is what everyone will experience. Everything you see in the world is created by the beliefs of the people who live here. In essence, it is beliefs that hold this reality together like a cosmic glue and determines exactly what you see.

I would highly recommend the book by Dr. Bruce Lipton…The Biology of Belief. I know this information about aging may be new to your ears; however, you better get used to it because there are numerous things coming in the winds that are going to blow your mind as far as health and extending your life many years beyond what most people consider normal. Advancements in technology and a shift in consciousness will be able to significantly extend your life here on this planet.

You can begin shifting your mental programs about aging right now. Again, they are only beliefs and you can reprogram your mind for living an extended amount of years. Consider what science has discovered; that your cells are programmed to survive for an indefinite amount of time. Now couple this with the idea that your mind can literally cause your cells to age slower or faster depending upon what you believe. Yes, eating healthy and living a balanced life is part of extending your life years.

What if you were to change the subconscious programs running in your mind to ones that support a long and healthy life, say to the age of 200? Is this possible? You bet it is! Where's the proof you say? Well, have you ever met someone that looked much younger than their actual age? Of course you have, we have all met people like this. The question is: why do these people look so much younger than their actual age? Give Up? It is because of the way they live their lives and the beliefs they carry. They also have a positive perspective of themselves which in turn reflects this in their appearance. These feelings and upbeat attitude towards life helps create bio-chemicals that strengthen your immune system and nourishes your cells.

Imagine what can happen if you could introduce a mental program into your subconscious mind that says…I AM LIVING TO THE AGE OF 200. Very intriguing isn't it? So, what age are you going to live to?

How To Slow The Aging Process

You can easily slow your aging process down significantly. The key lies in living a balanced life and maintaining a clean inter-cellular environment. Living as stress free as possible is one of the best things you can do for your health and can do wonders at keeping you feeling and looking young. Resolving suppressed emotions can also work wonders at freeing up tension on your body and cells which in turn will help you to feel better and look younger. In fact, releasing held onto emotions can do more benefit to your health and how young you look than any anti-wrinkle cream.

Here is a little secret that the skin care product companies don't want you to know. The health of your skin is directly dependent upon the internal state of your cells. If you are toxic internally, then it doesn't matter what kind of lotion you use on your skin. Some of these skin products will help your skin to look better; however, it is only a short term effect. If you want permanent results for younger looking skin then the key is to detoxify your cells and maintain this clean internal cellular environment. You can also experience dramatic results in younger looking skin by keeping your body properly hydrated. Water is of key importance to have your cells properly hydrated not only for overall health but for skin elasticity and softness. Most skin disorders are from lack of hydration and a toxic inter-cellular environment.

Holistic Health Practice:

Go to a place where you will not be disturbed. Sit or lie down and begin deep breathing. Take 10 deep breaths. Now, visualize yourself as looking younger than you are. Really feel what this is like. Bring in good feelings into this picture.

Say to yourself ..."I am living to the age of...put in the number of the age you want to live to. Now keep focusing on this number in your meditations. When you speak to others, tell them that you are going to live to this age. This belief will eventually enter into your subconscious mind. Notice the results in the coming months.

In order for this to be more effective it is advised to eat healthy and exercise. I highly recommend following my 8 Royal Diamonds of Optimum

Health. Combining both a shift in your consciousness and embodying the 8 Royal Diamonds into your life on a daily basis will work wonders at slowing your aging down. One other golden piece of information that will dramatically help slow your aging process is to live your passion. Living your passion creates so many life enhancing bio-chemicals in your body leaving you energized and invigorated. Follow these recommendations; your body will thank you. Try it and see. Let me know how it goes.

Your Body & Cells Already Hold The Fountain of Youth, You Just Have To Awaken To This Profound Truth!

Chapter 8

Silencing The Chattering Voice In Your Head

Did you ever wonder what your life would be like if you could turn that chattering voice off in your head? How peaceful and calm your life would be. Imagine how dramatically your life would change if you could find a way to reduce or stop the constant chirping in your mind?

Well, there is a way to at least reduce this constant bombardment of streaming thoughts. As I learned in life, you discover golden nuggets like this as you evolve and heal your being. Everyone who has ever existed on this planet has had to deal with their chattering mind. It is a normal part of our existence. If you are like most people, then you think that you are the only one that has this chattering mind. I used to think that I was the only one that had this constant chattering voice that never gave me any relief. Finally, I discovered a profound secret that worked very effectively at reducing and even stopping this nagging voice at times.

You see, as a child you get conditioned with all sorts of beliefs and opinions from society. Your family has the biggest impact on your mental conditioning. Hearing certain words and seeing certain life events over and over again become ingrained into your subconscious mind and serve as mental programs that run on autopilot without your conscious awareness. As you develop these mental programs in your childhood, you form certain beliefs about yourself and of life. You then start thinking you are these subconscious beliefs. Sooner or later you start acting out these mental programs or what I call wearing the masks of life. You literally act out the person you think you are. This person you think you are is an illusion.

This illusionary self is based upon the perceptions and beliefs you have formed from your environment such as family, friends, teachers and others in society. Humans wear these masks to ensure that they are loved and fit in. Little do we know that by wearing these masks and acting like someone other than our true inner being is harmful to our growth and development as children. This illusionary self takes on a personality of its own. You then start to believe everything this illusionary self tells you. As you do so, you steer further and further away from your true self.

This false self now becomes a major component of your being and acts like a dictator. This is how the chattering voice in your head takes control over you. On an unconscious level you have allowed a false personality to take over your being. At this point you think that there is nothing you can do to stop this chattering voice that runs continuously. This voice is judgmental, nagging, whining, complaining, demeaning, harsh and at times unreasonable causing you to act and speak unlike your true self. It has caused you a great deal of suffering over the years in the form of hardships and limitation. This voice is a saboteur (pronounced SAB-O-TOUR) meaning it sabotages almost all efforts by you to grow, evolve and express your true brilliance. This saboteur is your biggest obstacle in life for creating the magic you desire in the form of happiness, abundance, peace and joy. This saboteur is the real culprit to why you have not found peace or calm.

What is this saboteur? Some refer to it as the ego. This ego is much more powerful than you may think. It is the main cause for most of your suffering. As I have discovered you are suffering more from this chattering voice than anything else. Even physical pain is not as agonizing as your ego can be. The ego thrives on drama, chaos, heartache and misery. It literally uses these forms of life events as food at your expense. There are numerous tactics it uses to keep you locked in the illusion that you are your ego. The ego's biggest fear is that you will discover that you are not it. Thus, it does everything in its power to keep you locked in the illusion and lies. Your ego knows that if you discover the truth that you are not it, the ego would cease to exist.

Your ego is what separates you from the eternal SOURCE of all that is. When you equate yourself to be the ego, you severely limit your true potential. Thinking you are the ego, you feel disconnected, lonely, limited, fearful and lacking in self-esteem. Your ego wants you to think that everything in life should be hard and complex. It wants you bound by its erroneous concepts. After many years of equating yourself to be the ego, you become subconsciously addicted to chaos, drama, limitation and lack. Being in these vibrations only attracts to your life events that match this energy. This is exactly what your ego wants. It is like a grand buffet for your ego, all the while you suffer deep down inside.

Here is a secret that I learned on my path to self-awakening: You are a master. You have everything within you right now that you will ever need. The solutions to all of your life issues are deep within you and can be accessed any time. You are complete and whole as is. You require nothing to make you better. You were born in perfection and will always be perfect. The SOURCE of all that is only creates perfect things. Where humanity has gone wrong is that it has deviated from what the ONE has given. Humanity has gone wrong in consciousness and in doing so has separated itself from being firmly connected to the SOURCE.

Your ego wants you believing that you require things to make you better. The ego is a want-a-holic. It is never satisfied and never will be. It wants you in a constant want mode for in doing so keeps you locked in its grip. When you are in this state of consciousness you are not in your power and you are not being who you really are. In this state, your ego runs the show. This is sad because you are unconscious of this fact.

This is the exact state of many people on the earth. Their egos are running the show and they don't even know it. They think that they are consciously in control. This is part of the illusion. To remain in this state of unconsciousness will only attract more misery and heartache in your life. Haven't you proved this to yourself over and over again through the dramas in your life? It is ironic because a part of you actually likes these dramas. It is true. We have all at some time in our lives become addicted to misery on an unconscious level.

The truth is that you are powerful, you are whole and you are complete as you are. Your ego wants you thinking that you have to become greater than what you are. The second you think you require something to make you better; you separate yourself from the SOURCE and in doing so create chaos, drama and limitation in your life. The SOURCE only sends your way what you are vibrating out. The SOURCE of all that is only knows about beauty, abundance, peace and serenity, it knows nothing of the lack or limitation that you are vibrating.

The universe will only send to you life events that match your inner vibration. This is the universe's only way of communicating to you exactly what you are vibrating out. So, if you want to see where you are at in any aspect of your life then take a step back and look. The truth will be there. How are you relationships? How are your finances? How is your career? Is there anything that you can do about the chattering voice?

What I am about to reveal is of such profound importance for your overall wellbeing. This golden nugget of wisdom can help you in taking back your power from this illusionary personality. Are you ready to discover one of the simplest and yet most powerful ways to reduce and/or end the chattering voice in your head? How great is that going to be to actually take your power back from this personality that most people call the ego?

One of the easiest ways to begin taking your power back from your ego is to give it a name. You must separate yourself from the chattering voice in your head if you wish to have peace in life. This voice is not you. It is the YOU that you have created over the years in the forms of beliefs and perceptions. It is not real and only has life because you feed it every day by acting out this personality and listening to all the chattering in your head. So, go ahead and give it a name. Call it something pleasant such as a nickname you had when you were a child. You can even use a shortened version of your name. By doing this very simple process, you have just exposed your ego. It now knows that you know that you are not that voice.

Your ego has done everything in its power all these years to keep you from this knowledge. Now that you are conscious of this you easily can take your power back. So every time you hear the nagging, whining, judgmental, and mean voice coming out…simply pause and acknowledge it. Then say "I hear you ego but no thank you." Let it know that you are in control from now on. Be stern about it and really express this to your ego.

You will be amazed at the results you can experience by doing this simple exercise when you hear that chattering voice. One word of warning...your ego will attempt to trick you so you have to be very conscious of it at all times. It is funny how this illusionary personality will attempt to gain control back. You must remain steady and super conscious of this. Your ego is not at all as bad as some would have you believe. It is a part of being human and it simply requires that you learn to balance this aspect of your being into your psyche. Treat your ego as you would a child that requires direction and at times discipline.

Holistic Health Practice:

Another exercise you can do is to go into a deep meditation and call your ego out. Ask it what it wants. Have a regular conversation with it and see what it reveals.

You too can also discover important information from your ego. Be nice when approaching your ego. Talk to it as you would a friend. The last thing you want to do is approach your ego as an enemy. Be gentle and firm and let it know that you are the boss without being too forceful. Make sure you write down what your ego reveals so you can review it at later times. You will be amazed at what you discover. Try it and see.

You may not like what your ego reveals to you, however, you require knowing this information for taking your power back. As you become more conscious of what has been hidden from you, you will feel much better mentally, emotionally, physically and spiritually. As you begin to feel lighter and more peaceful your true inner self will reveal itself to you. It talks to you through your intuition and has a much different tone than your ego. Your true inner being is gentle, calm and loving. It is a complete opposite as far as personality goes. So, if you want to determine the voice that is talking to you is of your true inner self or that of your ego...simply notice the tone of the voice. If the voice is a tone of judgment, whining, complaining, negative and finding fault then you can be certain that it is your ego. If the voice is positive, loving, calm and gentle then it is of your True inner self.

Taking power back from your ego can free up so much energy and open so many doorways of opportunity that you will amazed. Your ego has caused you to use up so much energy in the form of hardships, emotional grief and limitation. It is time to free yourself and use that energy to create the life you truly desire. It all starts with the intention to take your power back. The question...do you choose to take your power back?

You Are A Divine Being And Are Perfect As Is. There Is No Need To Become More. You Are What You Seek And More Right Now. Awaken To This Truth!

Chapter 9

Discover Your Destiny, Be Healthy For Life!

There is within you a GIANT waiting for you to discover your life purpose. This GIANT waits anxiously and patiently for you to uncover the main reason you are here on this planet. You are here to fulfill a major life destiny. Discovering your life purpose is part of your evolution. In fact, when you live your passion and serve the role you are destined to, your life becomes magical.

How different would your life be if you lived your life with passion and fulfilled your destiny for being here on this planet? Do you honestly think you are here for no specific reason? The universe doesn't work that way. Once you discover your life purpose, you will never be the same again. Something I learned on my path to healing and discovering my life purpose is that it will require for you to step outside of your comfort zone. Your ideal life exists outside of the box you have created for yourself. This is where the happiness, joy, freedom, and abundance you seek lies. In essence, expanding into a bigger box is a shift in consciousness and can happen in a split second.

Fears and doubts can stop you from making this shift. Fear is only an illusion and yet can be responsible for keeping you inside your little box. You may end up living a miserable life because you never get to experience the bliss of living your destiny. Fear and a lack of belief in yourself sabotage your dreams. When you hide behind fear, you never get to discover your true potential. Here is a secret I discovered on my path to self -awakening. Running from your fears is running farther and farther away from the life you truly desire.

To conquer any fear, you must run towards that fear. It is the golden key to transmute any blocking fear. As you run toward your fear, you will realize that it is only an illusion and that on the other side awaits your life of bliss. It is all simply a choice. Simply choosing to go through your fears will open a new world to you. Deep down inside your soul constantly longs for expression. Follow this inner feeling for it will direct you to your life purpose. This is the only way your soul will be satisfied. It is the only way for you to experience the power you hold deep inside your being.

How To Discover Your Life Purpose

Perhaps you are not sure what your life purpose is? It is perfectly fine to go through periods of uncertainty. Something I learned is that your life interests will point you in the direction of what your life purpose is. I also believe the universe helps you to uncover your life purpose by sending specific life events your way.

Your life's most challenging times contain the biggest rewards within them. You too have a life purpose which entails helping the world in some manner.

When you help others, you get a feeling that cannot be described in words. Your whole body vibrates in a whole new way and physically you feel alive and energized. You feel is as if you are reborn. Look at people who you know are living their life passion. They look younger than what their real age is and they have so much energy. People who are living their passion are magical people. They are unstoppable and create amazing products and services that help humanity.

My question to you is…what is stopping you from living your life passion? Is it fear? You are not the only one since fear affects almost every single person on the path to self-awakening and self-discovery. Honor the fear for now and then choose to go beyond that illusionary thought form. Fear is only a thought and nothing else.

Holistic Health Practice:

A simple exercise you can do to uncover your life purpose is to write down what you are interested in. What brings you joy, what makes your heart sing? What would your ideal life be like if you could wave a wand and have it come true? Write this down. You will eventually discover what you are meant to do if you remain open and have the intention to do so. Here is a secret: The universe is waiting for you to show it that you are ready to live your passion. It all starts with a choice, a choice to evolve and grow into a bigger box. This means that you have to BE a new person. It is as simple as a shift in your consciousness. As you live your passion you will feel mentally, emotionally, physically and spiritually so much better. It is like a shot of adrenaline that propels you to a whole new life…the life you truly desire!

MAKE YOUR DESTINY, DON'T LET DESTINY MAKE YOU!

Rino

Chapter 11

Words of Wisdom To Lead You On Your Path To Health and Wellness

I wanted to leave you with some words of spiritual wisdom that I have learned in going through my experience with life in general. It is amazing how life teaches you important life lessons through your tribulations. What I have learned in life is that everything that happens in your life is there for expanding your consciousness and making you aware of who you really are. Things just don't happen to you; although that is what your EGO wants you to think.

We live in a world of cause and effect. Science has proven this many times over. Every life situation comes to teach you something. The funny thing is that most of the hardest times in your life contain the biggest lessons and the biggest rewards. Some people do not see the lessons and gifts in each life circumstance. It seems that some people want to have the tough times simply disappear.

Life doesn't work that way. No one gets to have life easy even though our egos want us to think that our lives are the toughest. This is an illusion. In fact, most of your worries are only illusions. Your fears, your doubts and your insecurities are all illusions. Most of these things have no validity and yet you act as if they are true. Realize that you are a master. You are a co-creator with the Infinite Spirit that created you and the entire universe. You may not believe this, however, it is absolutely true. You have and will continue to create most things that enter into your life. These events don't just happen to you. You are responsible for them. You are the one who sets up the frequency to attract these events to you, be it mainly on a subconscious level.

You see, your creator gave you free will and with this comes power. This power can be used to create great a life of bliss or one of chaos, drama and misery. You decide with your thoughts and feelings what you create in your life. At any moment in time you have an unlimited number of choices. With choices come consequences be they good or bad. It seems that some people simply refuse to believe that they are responsible for most of the circumstances that happen in their lives. They instead choose to believe that they have been dealt a bad deck of cards, had an unloving mother, an abusive father, a poor upbringing, a lack of education, little resources and on and on. They think that because of someone or something that this is why their lives are like this.

This mentality is playing the victim. We have all played the victim in our lives. Why? Most of us have been conditioned to react this way. It is much easier to put the blame on someone or something else than to stand up and assume responsibility for our own lives. It's much easier to play small than to break free from the bonds of limitation that society conditions us with. It is much easier to follow than to lead. It is much easier to feel inferior than feel powerful. Most people are scared to death of their true potential, their shining light.

So, out of fear people hide in their misery and in their shells that they have created throughout the years. They hide behind their masks and play those parts perfectly. They assume roles that they are not really comfortable with. They seek to please others more than they seek to please themselves. People do things just to fit in so they can feel wanted and appreciated. People at times stoop very low simply to get an ounce of recognition. People behave this way because they feel not good enough, smart enough, attractive enough, or deserving enough. People become different from their true selves just so they can feel a part of this world; so they don't go crazy.

Here is a secret for you: From the day you were born, you were perfect. In fact, there is perfection underneath all the masks and roles that you now play. The Infinite Spirit that created all that is only creates perfect things. You are perfect as is. There is no need to become more than what you already are. It is this constant striving to become more and to fit in that creates all your tribulations. The second you think you need something to make you better, you separate yourself from the source. And because you separate yourself, you become less powerful. Feeling less powerful you now attract more hard times in your life. These hard times are there to get your attention. They are screaming…YOU ARE OFF COURSE!

And because you don't hear or see these loud messages screaming to get back on course, you continue to veer farther and farther from your true self. You get so far away from your true self that when you look into the mirror, you no longer know who you are. You see a complete stranger, a foreigner. It is at this point where you feel lost, confused and alone that your biggest lesson of life is waiting. What is that lesson? That you are already perfect and that you need nothing to make you better. You are already whole, a complete package. You have strived to achieve and be more for so many years, when the whole time you were already perfect.

Life is ironic and comical, really. Here we are born powerful, perfect and whole. Yet, we go through life playing small. We hide behind fear and doubt our true potential. We fear so much what will happen when we bust through our reality box that we have confined ourselves in.

People feel powerless and inferior and thus create drama and chaos in their lives. They have to feed the illusion so they do everything possible to stay distracted and occupied. Because they feel un-whole they seek partners to wrap themselves with. They think that this will solve their loneliness and the emptiness that they feel inside. Then after some time when their partner no longer seem to fill the void inside, they shout, they blame and come to believe that it's all their fault for why the relationship has failed.

Life is a mystery, this is quite clear. It's all a state of consciousness. The emptiness and void that you feel deep down inside is really the peace and tranquility you seek. Many people seek to find peace and tranquility when the whole time is it right there under their nose. People tend to be scared of this emptiness and so flee from it, hide from it and distract themselves from it. It is unknown to us so that is why we fear this void so much. However, it is our true home, the place from where we came. It is the place we shall return once this game is over.

Your life tribulations you are experiencing are a manifestation of the power you possess. Do you now see how powerful you really are? It's not good or bad, it just is. Imagine if you can learn how to direct this power in the correct manner. The same way you used this awesome power to create drama and misery, you can now redirect this power to create beauty, peace and health. Again, it is all a state of consciousness. For there to be issues in your life it means that you had to plant seeds of disharmony, there is no other way. The common saying of You Shall Reap What You Sow applies here. When you plant seeds of drama, you will get drama. It is that simple. However, now you can start again and plant a new garden, one with seeds of health and beauty. Your garden will adapt to any seeds you plant. So, the question is... what seeds will you plant from now on?

To Your Health,

Rino Soriano

You may visit Rino's website to learn more about his coaching services, classes, speaking events and seminars. You can also learn more about holistic health products and supplements for helping you to live a healthy and conscious lifestyle. **Please www.RinoSoriano.com**

You can visit Amazon.com to view and purchase Rino's other books:

The Youngevity Revolution: The 12 Secret Spirals to Enduring Youth and Longevity

Why America Is Fat, The Truth Is Finally Revealed

Sensational Slimming Secrets, A Revolutionary Pathway To A Healthier and Slimmer You

Mystic Smoothies: The 33 Most Delicious & Nutritious Smoothies To Rock The Planet

Fun Food Fantastic: Knock Your Socks Off Meal Creations

Consciousity: The Crystalline Key For Transforming Planet Blue

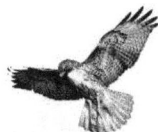

Produced By Flying Hawk Productions™

www.ingramcontent.com/pod-product-compliance
Lightning Source LLC
Chambersburg PA
CBHW050119280326
41933CB00010B/1167